Breezing Through Menopause:
A Holistic Doctor's Customized Approach to Hormonal Change

By Dr Suzanne Ciotti

Copyright © 2020 by Suzanne Ciotti M.D.
All rights reserved
ISBN-9798640453102

Table of Contents

Chapter ONE: *Changes During Menopause* — Page 4

Chapter TWO: *Perimenopause* — Page 10

Chapter THREE: *Inflammation and Menopause* — Page 19

Chapter FOUR: *Weight Gain and Menopause* — Page 23

Chapter FIVE: *Vaginal Care and Sex* — Page 30

Chapter SIX: *Menopause and Your Bones* — Page 38

Chapter SEVEN: *Thyroid Issues in Menopause* — Page 44

Chapter EIGHT: *Menopause and Your Brain* — Page 52

Chapter NINE: *Hormonal Treatment Approach to Menopause* — Page 57

Chapter TEN: *Non-Hormonal Treatment for Menopause* — Page 69

Chapter ELEVEN: *Putting It All Together, An Intentional Living Plan* — Page 76

Who Has Time for Menopause?

Perimenopause occurs at an incredibly challenging time for many women as changes are commonly happening in the body, home and career. For some women during their 50s, work may become more demanding as they advance in their field, or they may seek a new career entirely. They may be experiencing their children moving to college, or older parents who are faced with disability and can no longer live independently. Internally, they may be experiencing physical, unpredictable changes in the way their body and mind looks and functions. Prior to this time of life, the responsibilities of child raising, working full time, or just making ends meet may have strengthened their role as the stable, predictable rock of the family or community. For many women, it has been an all-out endeavor leaving them drained but fulfilled, living a full life, balancing family, jobs, education and volunteer work. Perhaps this is true for you. As you enter this new phase of life, ripe with possibility, you may strive for stability and predictability or something else entirely. Possibly as your kids leave the nest for college, jobs and travel, you desire to dig deeper into your demanding job, or start a new career or hobby. How ironic that during this time of external change women also experience the internal, unpredictable changes of menopause, accompanied by hot flashes, sleepless nights and brain fog. With this book I hope to shed some light on these internal, biological changes that women face during midlife by using a comprehensive, holistic approach in which I will explain the biology behind those changes and offer a variety of options for treatment and management.

The topic of menopause, with its biological changes, typically catches women off guard. When does it begin? What are the typical symptoms? Will I need to take medications or can I handle this on my own? What would be the side effects of starting a new hormonal therapy or not starting therapy? While discussing options for management, it often becomes apparent that a better understanding of the physiological changes that are occurring would help a women to understand if treatment is necessary. Often this discussion with their physician includes considerations regarding symptoms, risk factors and goals, as well as education of basic physiological changes of menopause. There is often not enough time during a typical office visit to provide this in-depth information to help a women make the best choice regarding hormone therapy. This is why this book was born: to provide a larger discussion of considerations during menopause.

As mentioned previously, menopause comes at a chaotic time for women. For a few lucky women the transition is seamless for the most part: periods stop, they may have a few hot flashes and that is it. But for many women, it is a Pandora's box of unpredictable symptoms that no one had warned them about. As physicians, we do not receive medical training about the myriad of menopausal symptoms. However, over the years of clinical practice, many physicians note that there is a catalogue of diverse symptoms in patients including hot flashes, night sweats, insomnia, depression, anxiety, mental fogginess, joint pain, vaginal dryness, rapid heart rate, dry skin, brittle hair, fatigue, decreased libido, visual changes and weight gain (especially centrally). For many patients, it is also a time when some medical conditions seem to be newly expressed, like hypo/hyperthyroid, hypertension and the onset of osteoporosis. For a woman in midlife, it may appear that their body has become unpredictable. It can be a very frightening time. Is this the beginning of getting old and losing one's health? Will I ever be the same? How long will this last? Having the knowledge of what symptoms are related to menopause and what you can do about them can be very empowering. I hope this book will provide some assurance there is an end in sight, even if you choose to ride it out. There are many tools that you can use to stay healthy and functional normally in menopause. I would even challenge women to use this as an opportunity to be healthier and more self-aware than they have ever been.

Each woman is very different in their personal experiences during this transition, and treatment options need to be individualized based on those symptoms the patient is experiencing and medical conditions providers may be treating. There is no "one size fits all". When a woman comes into the office, they generally have a suspicion that something is not quite right with their hormones. Generally they have already done a lot of their own investigation, talking to family members and friends, or researching online. Often they will bring a book on menopause that seemed to strike a chord for them and helped to explain some of their symptoms. Perhaps they know other women who have very strong opinions about hormonal treatment both good and bad. It is very important during this initial conversation to discuss one's fears and desires during this transition so that the appropriate screening and treatment can be made together with their provider.

In the next few chapters, I will draw on both clinical experience and recent scientific evidence, when available. I will guide you through an overview of hormones throughout a women's lifecycle and into perimenopause and menopause. We will look at hormonal and non-hormonal treatment options and which ones have worked best for patients for different conditions in menopause and perimenopause. In later chapters, I will discuss how hormones influence specific parts of the body, such as bones and vaginal health. I will emphasize the importance of treatment options that are individualized, taking into consideration personal medical history, family history, symptom management and possible side effects. This concise guide is designed to be used as a reference as you make choices regarding your care.

Chapter One:
Changes During Menopause

> Sigourney Weaver said, "When you're young, there's so much now that you can't take it in. It's pouring over you like a waterfall. When you're older, it's less intense, but you're able to reach out and drink it. I love being older."
> *Esquire*, January 2010

Let's start with a simplified introduction to a woman's hormones over their lifespan, since it is these hormonal changes that influence a woman's experience of menopause, primarily a significant drop in estrogen. Hormones are "chemical messengers" that are secreted in small amounts into the blood stream to signal our organs to act a certain way. They very powerfully influence our body and brain, which we will specifically discuss in the next chapters. The major sex hormones, estrogen, progesterone and testosterone, are produced by the ovaries during a woman's childbearing years. During puberty, a female teenager's ovaries are stimulated by the pituitary gland in the brain to activate the ovaries. This begins a complex, synchronized rise and fall of hormones, primarily progesterone and estrogen, during a typical menstrual cycle that will continue over the next 30-40 years until menopause. In a typical menstrual cycle, estrogen peaks in the middle of a cycle, stimulating the ovaries to release an ovum or egg. Where the egg was released in the ovary there is a "shell" left behind; this is called the corpus luteum. This will produce a hormone called progesterone that stimulates the uterine lining so that the uterus may provide a rich, nutritive environment for the potential fertilized egg or embryo. If a woman does not become pregnant during her cycle, the hormone progesterone falls, resulting in stimulation of a period or uterine bleeding. This menstrual cycle is represented by the following graph:

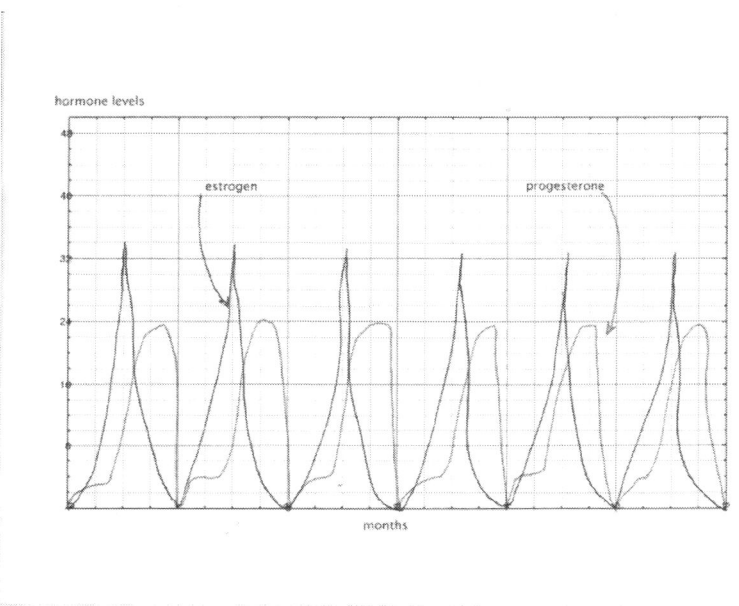

Regular Menstrual Cycles

This cyclical production of hormones results in a predictable pattern of periods that occur about every 28 days on average. The hormones produced will circulate throughout the body to affect nearly every cell. To put it another way, throughout a menstrual cycle, a woman's body is preparing for a potential pregnancy. This is why each cycle, a woman will feel like they would in early pregnancy with breast tenderness and fatigue, commonly referred to as premenstrual syndrome.

As we get into our forties, the ovaries work less efficiently, making lower amounts of progesterone at times. Women may also experience lack of ovulation altogether, resulting in months between periods, or spotting between periods. The pattern of estrogen and progesterone during this phase looks something like this:

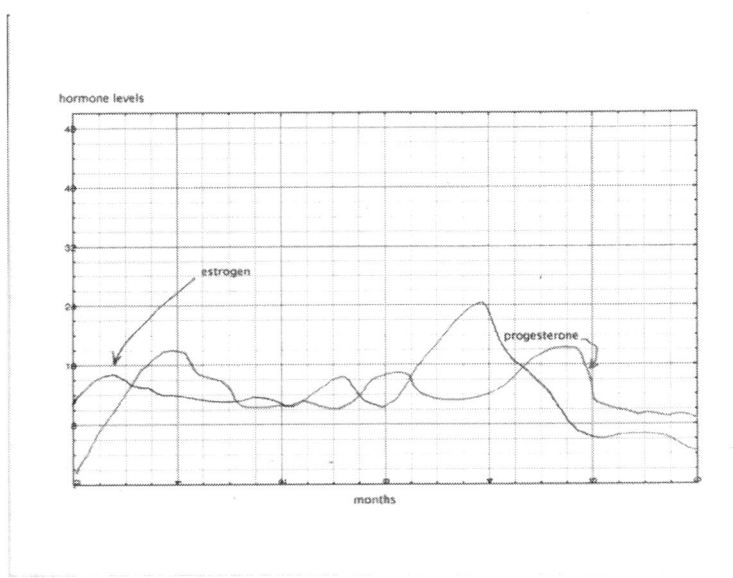

Perimenopause

For many women during this phase, each cycle feels different and unpredictable, sometimes causing bloating, moodiness and irregular periods. We will come back to a discussion of symptoms and treatments for this phase in the next chapter, exclusively dedicated to perimenopause.

During menopause, the ovaries will stop working altogether, causing a decline in estrogen, progesterone and testosterone to nearly immeasurable levels. The timing of this typically occurs between 45-55 years of age and will peak around 51. This results in low levels of estrogen, progesterone and testosterone. This can be graphically represented this way (y-axis hormone levels):

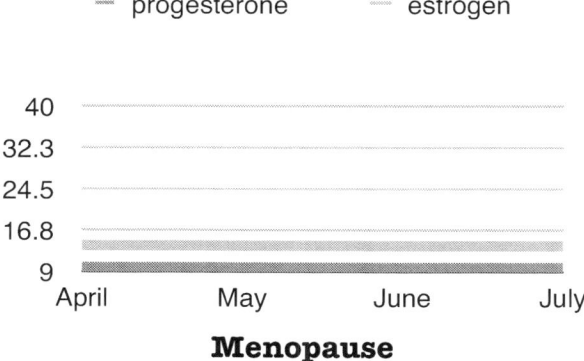

Menopause

This pattern results in no periods. We typically define menopause when a woman has gone a year without a period. Less well defined, perimenopause is considered the time prior to menopause when a woman is experiencing unpredictable cycles. Next let's discuss what symptoms and bodily changes occur when estrogen drops to low levels, as seen during menopause.

Like most hormones, it can be surprising to learn that nearly every cell in our body is influenced by estrogen, and the symptoms are varied among individuals. However, not all women have all the symptoms, and some women are fortunate enough to have NO symptoms of menopause. Because of this, each woman needs to be clear with their provider about what symptoms they are having and for how long—include all your symptoms even if you are not sure they are related to menopause. As we will discuss in the next chapters, there are many symptoms and medical conditions that are influenced by the changes brought on by menopause. Sharing your experience and concerns with your provider will help you determine if hormonal therapy is the right choice for you.

If you are a woman going through menopause currently, you probably have already experienced the most common symptom of menopause: hot flashes. It is also the most reliable indication, next to periods stopping, that you are in menopause. Hot flashes can occur during the day or night, often interrupting sleep. Hot flashes commonly start in the chest, neck and temples and spread outwardly making a woman flush and feel sweaty, like stepping into a sauna. It seems for a majority of women that hot flashes peak from three to nine months after the last period and gradually get less frequent and less severe over time. Some women will continue to have occasional hot flashes for the next five years, triggered by emotions, alcohol, smoking and hot environment. For most women, hot flashes will stop after five years, but for some (less than one percent of women), hot flashes may last a lifetime.

Hot flashes are triggered by the brain sensing lower estrogen, increasing the secretion of lutenizing hormone (LH) and follicle stimulating hormone (FSH), "messengers" that stimulate ovary function. When the ovaries stop functioning, the hormones FSH and LH increase in the blood stream and can be measured in a common blood test to determine if menopause has occurred. In addition, because hot flashes are related to estrogen withdrawal, they can also be triggered by sudden cessation of estrogen replacement therapy such as estrogen pills. This is why physicians usually suggest that estrogen is tapered slowly so that hot flashes can be avoided. Estrogen therapy usually works very well to stop or lessen hot flashes, and because of this, hot flashes are usually easy to treat.

Night sweats are actually somewhat different than hot flashes, although they can occur at the same time for some women during menopause. Night sweats can occur in both women and men and appear to occur when the body is under stress, such as cancer, menopause or autoimmune disorders. They also occur with some medications, like antidepressants and diabetes medications. Often women in their forties will present to the office describing night sweats and not hot flashes. They will describe "waking up drenched in sweat." Years just prior to menopause (perimenopause), a woman is experiencing changes in hormones that are at suboptimal levels, and they may frequently experience night sweats.

There are other less well-known symptoms of menopause: arthritis, tachycardia, changes in concentration, insomnia, dry skin, hair loss, weight gain (typically in a central or abdominal pattern), lack of libido, anxiety, depression, urinary symptoms and vaginal dryness. Arthritis, or painful joints, may present at the time of menopause and can often be less painful with estrogen replacement therapy (ERT); this will be discussed in Chapter Three. Vaginal dryness typically starts a few years after a woman's last period and will be discussed in Chapter Five. Mood related symptoms such as anxiety and depression may start during perimenopause or menopause and may be related to the lack of concentration and trouble multitasking that many women describe during menopause. Insomnia may occur with hot flashes and result in trouble falling asleep or staying asleep. We will learn exciting research on how decreased estrogen affects the brain in Chapter Ten.

As part of the evaluation of menopause treatment, having your list of symptoms with an understanding of how much they affect your daily life will help dictate the best options for treatment during your discussion with your healthcare provider. As you read the next chapters, reflect on your current medical issues so that you can determine if they may have started at the same time as menopause. This will help your provider determine if menopause considerations may be beneficial to support healing and balance in those medical conditions that may otherwise have been thought of as separate from menopause.

Chapter Two: Perimenopause

For some women, the years prior to menopause are the most challenging, even more so than complete menopause. For a woman in her 30s or 40s, this may be frequent, heavy periods that are longer and more painful than thos during her 20s. The periods may occur closer together, rather than getting less frequent, as one might predict. A woman may also experience night sweats, worsened moods and trouble sleeping. These symptoms are generally due to poor ovarian function or aging ovaries. Some months the ovaries may make an egg and sometimes they stay dormant. It may also mean that even during the months that an egg is made, the corpus luteum is not making progesterone quite as effectively, a very common deficiency in perimenopause. Recognizing the hormonal changes during this phase of life helps to determine what treatments may be best for you. This chapter, we will also explore common hormonal syndromes that women may experience during the premenopausal years.

As you may remember from the previous chapter, here is an chart of the moon-inspired rhythm of hormones for most women in their 20s-30s month to month:

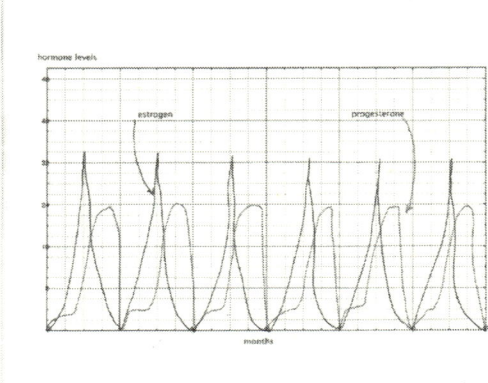

And here is an example of hormonal changes got women in their 40s-50s month to month:

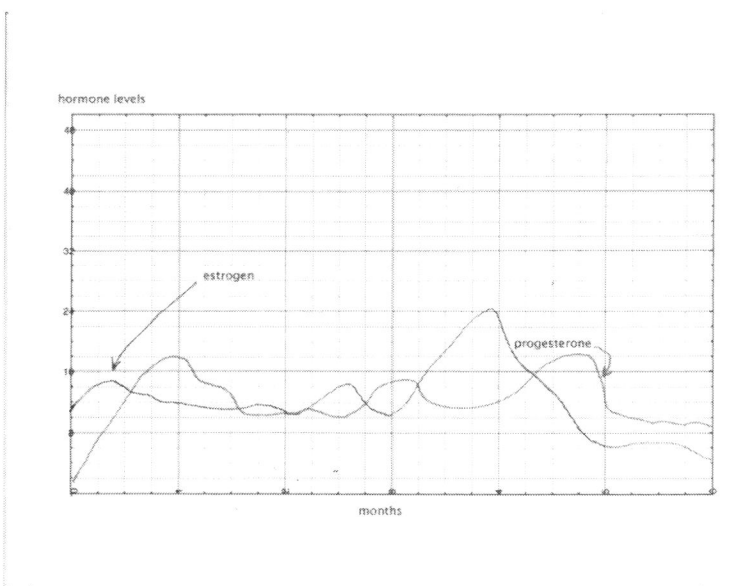

As you can see, one is predictable and represents the complex coordinated choreography between the ovaries, uterus and pituitary gland—it is a beautiful dance of hormone feedback loops and rhythms. As women age, there are problems with coordination of hormones resulting in unpredictable highs and lows of estrogen and progesterone. This causes challenges for many women and clinicians identifying where a woman is in their hormonal cycle during any day of the month so that they can understand why they may feel more bloated or moody. With menopause your ovaries STOP and we can replace what is not being made. However, in perimenopause, one day hormones may be very high and seven days later they have dropped. There is no consistency or predictability cycle to cycle, making it difficult to determine hormone deficiencies with a blood test.

For providers, determining if symptoms of perimenopause are definitively related to hormonal changes has several challenges. First, hormonal levels vary day to day and are unpredictable. In order to understand a woman's pattern we would have to measure hormone levels every day, which is not practical for most women. Secondly, if this was accomplished, the same pattern may not occur the next month (remember our lack of pattern on our charts during perimenopause). Thirdly, there are wide ranges of normal for each phase in a woman's cycle, so hormone levels are typically low just after a period and increase just prior to a period. In addition there are no published guidelines for what hormone levels should be in order to treat certain symptoms of perimenopause—more research is needed.

However, we do get clues to what might help a patient by extrapolating from timing of symptoms that a woman has during her cycle. When cycles are predictable, symptoms can be related to hormones if they occur cyclically (usually every month). For example, some women experience increased moodiness just prior to their period and this occurs predictably on the 25th day of her cycle. For the woman experiencing perimenopause, there are many possible symptoms: feelings of irritability, fatigue or difficulty sleeping certain months and not others. You may have more breast tenderness at times, or night sweats for several evenings. Also common are periods that are closer together and heavier, sometimes even resulting in low iron or anemia. Some symptoms may be related to low estrogen and others to low progesterone.

Low Estrogen States

As a woman approaches the average menopause age of fifty, they may miss periods for several months and then have a heavy, random period while on vacation. If periods stop for a few months, they may even have hot flashes that typically signal menopause. The hot flashes may even go away completely just prior to their period. This is because the ovaries are making follicles and eggs very sporadically and will release a pulse of estrogen—just as if hormone replacement had been started. This pulse of estrogen suppresses hot flashes. However, during each missed ovulation when estrogen levels naturally drop, the cycle of hot flashes comes back very strong. In other words, women in this pattern are constantly going through a cycle of estrogen withdrawal, with the corresponding hot flashes and sleep disturbances.

Theoretically, if we were to stop having periods and stop making estrogen definitively, we could go through the most intense time of hot flashes, usually about six to 12 months and be done with it. It is the WITHDRAWAL from hormones that seems to cause the most disruption to our bodies during perimenopause. But do not despair! Armed with this knowledge, we can devise a plan for tackling the life disruption of perimenopause. Sometimes suppressing our ovaries from making a random follicle and egg every 3-6 months is the key—this is usually done with hormones described below. We can also decide to use non-hormonal herbals or medications for the years that hormones are fluctuating widely to help restore balance emotionally and physically. Sometimes just the knowledge that this will not last forever is helpful to management and brings hope to many patients.

In addition to periodically experiencing low estrogen levels, women in perimenopause may have low progesterone.

Low Progesterone States

As discussed previously, progesterone is a lovely hormone produced by the corpus luteum during the the last half of a woman's cycle, also call the follicular phase. It helps the lining of the uterus become soft and filled with life-sustaining nutritive blood for a developing fetus. For a woman, it is a "feel-good hormone" in some respects, providing help with sleep and a sense of calmness. For many women, it is the lack of progesterone just prior to a period that will cause moodiness, insomnia and mental fogginess. It also causes small blood vessels in the uterine lining to contract and release prostaglandins involved in the sensation of cramping prior to a period. Once recognized and determined with blood testing, progesterone can be supplemented several ways to relieve symptoms. Prescription progesterone may have a few negative effects. It can stimulate appetite and increase breast tenderness—after all, it is a hormone responsible for getting a woman's body ready for potential pregnancy. However, progesterone supplementation tends to be safer and comes with less side effects than estrogen-based treatments.

Evaluation and Treatment of Progesterone Defect

Some women determine they have a lack of progesterone hormone while being evaluated for infertility even as young as 20-30 years of age. This "luteal phase defect" may be treated with progesterone by a fertility specialist during days 14-28 to help a women sustain a pregnancy. For a women interested in knowing if progesterone may be causing perimenopausal symptoms, progesterone levels can be measured on day 20 of her cycle, usually with a common blood test.

Progesterone can then be supplemented during the luteal phase, which is day 14-28 in a typical cycle. There are several forms of progesterone to chose from. Prometrium 100 mg or 200 mg may be used, which is a standard prescription that can be obtained by a regular pharmacy with a provider's authorization. Also available is compounded micronizide progesterone, which can be made in any dosage—usually 25 mg to 400 mg for treatment of low progesterone in the luteal phase. This prescription must be obtained from a compounding pharmacy. There are also several progesterone-like supplements: wild yam cream, evening primrose oil 2-4 grams a day, Vitex (chastetree berry) 20-40 mg a day and micronized progesterone cream five to 100 mg a day.

Another option for management is to take the progesterone every day and not just on days 14-28 of your cycle. Sometimes we will adjust to a higher dose of progesterone when a woman is closer to her period. This is particularly helpful for women who have very irregular periods. Taken this way, progesterone may suppress a woman's ovaries and help keep hormones more stable day to day. Using progesterone in any of the forms listed is very low in side effects while perhaps alleviating symptoms of PMS or perimenopause.

Estrogen and Contraceptive Treatment Options

Another, more traditional way to treat perimenopause is to stop the ovaries from ovulating completely using hormonal birth control measures. This approach works by smoothing out hormonal fluctuations and, therefore, the symptoms caused by fluctuating hormones. For many women, this has been the only option offered to them by their providers and is commonly used. It may be a good option for many women and is especially helpful when periods are very heavy, frequent and painful. This includes birth control pills, patches, and rings; the hormonal IUDs (intrauterine devices); nexplanon progesterone inserts; and Depoprovera injections. Women considering these options should keep in mind that there are many forms of birth control, and we can work to find the one that is right for the individual. Over the past 15 years, birth control pills have been formulated with significantly less hormones, potentially decreasing side effects for some women.

In this category, many women do well with the progesterone containing IUD, such as Mirena or Liletta. As mentioned before, progesterone helps stabilized the uterine lining resulting in cessation of periods. It also helps suppress wild hormonal swings of perimenopause. In addition, it is very good for pregnancy prevention during this time of life—more effective than birth control pills, and the risk of blood clot formation is not near the level of estrogen-containing birth control pills. For these reasons, many women find that an IUD may help with the menopausal transition. In fact, an IUD may be so effective at decreasing menopause symptoms that a woman may not realize that they are going through menopause because their periods have stopped as a result of the hormonal IUD. Menopause can be determined by the following protocol in this situation: if a woman starts to have hot flashes, add estrogen replacement at a low dose until the IUD is at the end of its six-year lifespan. At this point the IUD can be removed and the provider can test hormones (typically FSH) several months after removal to confirm menopause.

Magnesium Supplementation

Magnesium is a special, ubiquitous mineral—one can argue that explanation of its benefits deserve its own book. Briefly, magnesium it a fantastic mineral found abundantly in all green plants, and humans probably don't get as much as they should. Adding magnesium to your daily routine at 250 mg-1000 mg at bedtime is very useful for sleep and for relaxing muscles. It is particularly useful for menstrual cramps, and can be taken once a day at 250-500 mg as long as cramps are problematic—even if only one day a month. It is a powerful smooth-muscle relaxer (which is, after all, what the uterus is) and is very effective. The recommended approach is to start on the lower end of 250 mg of magnesium oxide once at bedtime and increase as needed up to 1250 mg. Beware that if you start too high, you may experience diarrhea. As an aside, taking magnesium is helpful during times when you are more prone to constipation, such as during travel, and is very convenient since it is in tablet form.

Polycystic Ovarian Syndrome

Polycystic Ovarian Syndrome may cause some challenges when trying to regulate hormones in the perimenopausal woman and deserves some additional recommendations. Polycystic ovarian syndrome (PCOS) for a long time has been considered a triad of symptoms including acne and increased facial hair, a tendency to form cysts on the ovaries with irregular periods, and pre-diabetes or in high-insulin state. In the past it was thought to be related to obesity; currently, we understand that even women with normal weight can have this syndrome. It can occur at any age from puberty to menopause. It is often difficult to diagnose since there is not one specific blood test and may go unrecognized for some individuals. For these women, it appears that the addition of a medication for regulation of glucose called metformin actually helps regulation of periods and glucose metabolism. It may also help with fertility for many women unable to get pregnant. Sometimes the medication spironolactone, a testosterone receptor blocking medication, will be used for these women to combat facial hair, and acne.

Recommendations for treatments for menopause/perimenopause mentioned in this book may also be used, such as determining progesterone status or use of herbals. In addition, women with PCOS with or without obesity should be encouraged to have a diet without excessive carbohydrates in order to discourage a hyper-insulin state in the body, thought to stimulate the ovaries to produce large cysts. Recognition of this syndrome early for women is very helpful since a diet low in carbohydrates may also help slow the progression to diabetes in their lifetime.

There are other endocrine disorders that may cause irregular periods that are not directly related to changes in estrogen or progesterone, such as thyroid disorder. Also, women who are obese may have stores of estrogen in their adipose or fat tissue. This may cause irregular or heavy periods. It is important to work with a knowledgeable physician in investigating these causes. Keep in mind that depression, anxiety and a high-stress lifestyle can also make periods irregular or could cause missed periods as well. There is a section in this book outlining strategies for regulation of sleep and mood since this is especially important in menopause, but has a role in all phases of life as well.

Evaluation of irregular periods prior to menopause should initially include a physical exam by a healthcare provider, including a pap smear. It may be necessary to check a pelvic ultrasound for structural abnormalities such as benign uterine fibroids or ovarian cysts. Cervical cultures are likely to be performed. Keeping up with your routine, preventative medical care will help maintain your health during this challenging time.

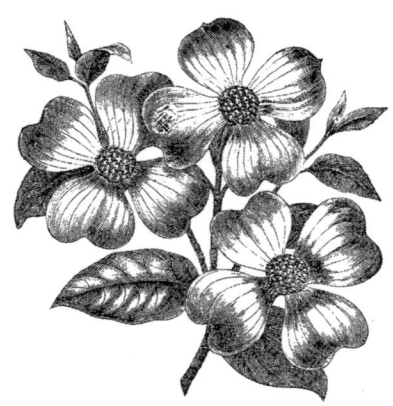

Chapter Three:
Inflammation and Menopause

It may come as no surprise that medical research has just recently started to recognize that there are differences in the way men and women should be studied in formal, scientific trials. Changes in the sex hormones over the life of an individual for both men and women and their effects on different disease states are starting to attract attention in scientific research possibly due to interest in "anti-aging" medicine. This new research suggests that the months and years just after menopause seem to encourage inflammation at a very cellular level involving arteries, joints and even the brain. We will discuss next an what medical conditions seem to be worsened by our hormonal changes and their effects on menopause and review new research investigating these changes. Included are theories suggesting the mechanism these hormonal changes have at a cellular level. We will also review specific autoimmune diseases that may be affected. Knowledge of these changes may help the reader understand why your specific conditions may be exacerbated by hormonal changes, such as arthritis, lupus, allergies, vasculitis, kidney disease or autoimmune hepatitis.

There are several inflammatory conditions that tend to develop during menopause that are not well recognized by many physicians, namely Hashimoto's thyroiditis, worsening of inflammatory arthritis, multiple sclerosis, and other autoimmune diseases. What is an autoimmune disease? An autoimmune disease by definition is when the body's immune system attacks an individual's very own normal cells. Typically, our immune system is designed to stop infection from viruses, bacterial and fungus that cause infections in our body. However, in autoimmune disease, this system goes into overdrive resulting in damage to our organs. For example, in thyroiditis, the immune system is attacking the thyroid gland and in rheumatoid arthritis our body's natural inflammatory response is attacking part of our own DNA, which results in damage to the joints, skin and kidneys, primarily. The complete mechanism of why this occurs and why it is stimulated by hormones is not well known. There is growing evidence that supplementing estrogen will lessen this unwanted inflammatory response and activation of the immune system. Therefore, if you are newly diagnosed with an autoimmune illness at the same time you transition through menopause, hormone replacement therapy may be a consideration. We will review further recent scientific investigation that may shed some light on this correlation.

In a review by Desai MK and Brinton RD (2019) titled *Autoimmune Disease in Women: Endocrine Transition and Risk Across the Lifespan* published in the journal Frontiers in Endocrinology, the authors found that hormonal changes during a woman's lifetime were associated with the development of autoimmune disease during adolescence, pregnancy and menopause in many studies. They looked at type 1 diabetes, lupus, rheumatoid arthritis, multiple sclerosis and psoriasis and compared what happened to these diseases during puberty, pregnancy and menopause. Overall they found that women with type one diabetes had higher mortality than men overall, with more microvascular complications in women with premature menopause. They also found that in women with lupus, there were less flares of this disease post menopause, however there was more damage from each flare. For rheumatoid arthritis, there was more joint destruction post menopause, however, hormone replacement therapy had a protective effect. In addition, multiple sclerosis had a peak incidence in the post-menopause age group; psoriasis also had more exacerbations during the post menopausal time frame. They concluded that more studies will need to done that emphasized menopause and autoimmune disease.

Desai and Brinton suggest in their review of studies that there are several biological factors involved that need further study. These included changes in genetic expression of genes as well as an altered inflammatory response with increased activation of T-cell mediated immunity and changes in other chemicals involved in inflammation. They suggest that in addition to estrogen, progesterone and testosterone, other hormonal changes such as increasing prolactin and leptin may play a role as well as our microflora. They suggest that puberty, pregnancy and menopause provide the "tipping point" for exacerbation of autoimmune states due to the interplay of these mechanisms. In their article, they suggest that for some diseases estrogen therapy may be helpful, but additional studies for each autoimmune disease and the role of HRT will be needed.

In my own practice, women who suffer with joint pain that corresponds with the start of menopause may find pain improved by low doses of HRT fairly quickly, usually within three months. I was particularly interested in studies on the subject to help me in counseling patients. A review by Mitali Talsania titled *Menopause and Rheumatic Disease* from Rheum Dis Clin North Am in 2017 provided an overview of sparse studies on the subject. Her review suggests that women who have increased joint pain do not have evidence on x-ray that arthritis is lessened by taking estrogen therapy in the hands, but there may be a decrease in arthritis in large joints including the hips of up to 40 percent of women studied. In all studies, there is an association with increased arthritis postmenopause; however it is unclear if this association is related to aging and not to lower estrogen. More studies are needed on this subject; however, it may be worthwhile to try hormonal therapy if you suffer from severe joint pain that coincided with the start of menopause.

Other autoimmune disease that may be activated or worsened with menopause are diabetes, multiple sclerosis, lupus, rheumatoid arthritis, Sjogren's disease, autoimmune hepatitis and psoriasis. It is beyond the scope of this book to go into each disease state, however, autoimmune thyroiditis is discussed at length in chapter seven since it is more commonly seen. Of note, women make up 75 percent of people challenged with autoimmune disease overall, so hormonal influences are particularly important in this group. Women with a family history of autoimmune disease may have increased risk of activation of these diseases during menopause, so keep in mind your particular family history at this important life transition.

What is the takeaway from this complicated topic? Hormonal changes are an under-recognized factor in many diseases, specifically autoimmune diseases, which are traditionally very challenging to treat. Although much more research should be done, the addition of HRT or modification of HRT may need to be considered to help quality of life. Changes in diet and lifestyle may need to be implemented as well to help modulate inflammation in the body. In the last chapter, we will discuss a lifestyle plan that will help you on your quest for a healthy, increased quality of life which is designed to decrease inflammation in the body.

Chapter Four
Weight Gain and Menopause

Second to hot flashes, the next most common complaint of patients in menopause is this: "I've gained weight and it is mostly in my middle; I used to have a flat stomach!" Sound familiar? I live in the very active community of Durango, Colorado, and many of my patients are very weight conscious with healthy lifestyles involving outdoor exercise pursuits like biking, running, hiking and kayaking. Even for these active women, weight would increase during menopause with corresponding distribution in the abdomen or stomach area, despite having stable weight for years. Over time I realized that weight gain during menopause occurs for most women; but women may control how much weight is gained with diet and exercise. During menopause, keeping your weight stable and not increasing is an achievement. This challenge with weight gain peaks in the first few years after the start of menopause and returns to a new, more predictable normal after that time. Being aware of this phenomenon and diligently watching diet during this time may be the difference between gaining two or twenty-five pounds.

As you may know, it is healthy to maintain an ideal weight to decrease your risk of developing heart disease, strokes and diabetes. Unfortunately, in addition to weight gain, menopause is a time when many women find that their blood pressure is higher and cholesterol is higher, making them at increased risk for stroke and heart disease. This may be in part due to the inevitable weight gain of menopause and changes on the blood vessels as well as liver production of less healthy cholesterol (HDL cholesterol). It is well known that weight gain will increase blood pressure and cholesterol, and weigh loss can help control these conditions. Why do we develop high blood pressure as we age? There may also be a role of epigenetic factors in menopause causing activation of particular genes in our DNA. This is a new discipline in genetics which studies environmental factors that trigger the expression of our genes. It appears that there are many factors that may influence this DNA activation: environment, lifestyle, hormones and stress all play a role. More than likely, there is a significant role of hormonal changes and epigenetic factors; this may explain why some women experience hypertension, diabetes and high cholesterol without significant weight gain during menopause. Please see additional readings for a more in-depth overview of a recent look at this phenomena by Riya Kanherkan, et al. However, treatment of genetically triggered high blood pressure, diabetes and obesity still relies on the same modalities as traditional treatments, such as watching diet primarily and, if necessary, medications.

Because there are so many potential changes to different systems in a woman's body during menopause, it is very important to continue regular exams, blood work and screening tests during this time of life. This means seeing an internist or family practice doctor in addition to a gynecologist. In general, keeping track of weight gain during menopause will be a major factor in controlling your blood pressure and cholesterol during menopause and will decrease one's risk of heart disease and stroke. As we will discuss, controlling weight gain is incredibly challenging during menopause.

Overall it is difficult to understand the mechanism for weight gain and hormonal change, although there has been a recognized link between hormonal treatments and weight gain in better known cases. For example, progesterone (Megace) is prescribed in cancer patients to help increase appetite and promote weight gain. In addition some women find that hormonal contraception or birth control pills increased their weight. For women in menopause we know that estrogen and progesterone levels become very low but still there is weight gain. So which is it? Are higher or lower levels of estrogen, progesterone and testosterone influencing weight?

Recent obesity and weight management research shows just how complicated maintaining weight and losing weight can be during menopause. Some studies find that counting and limiting calories or carbohydrates may not be enough to help women effectively loose weight during this time. In fact, there are specific genes involved in determining our weight "set point." In addition, there may be a role of changing intestinal microbiome in maintaining weight. Studies find that adding probiotics to mice, such as lactobacillus, may help promote a healthy weight in controlled studies. Also, there is evidence that specific diets (those diets higher in protein and fiber) may help in the secretion of leptin and ghrelin, so that our appetite is decreased and we feel fuller faster. Another way to control these hormones of appetite, including brain derived growth factor, may be intermittent fasting, or not eating for 12-48 hours once or twice a week. This optimizes these appetite suppressing hormones for weight loss. Finding the proper lifestyle balance will take trial and error depending on the individual.

What is encouraging is that in the past few years there has been specific research on the topic of weight gain in menopause and if ERT is helpful. This important research on ERT and weight gain has developed in part because of our national obesity epidemic in the United States and the resulting higher incidences of diabetes, heart disease and liver disease in those with increased abdominal fat, the same pattern that occurs in menopause. Addressing weight gain in menopause is therefore very important and should be a goal when considering ERT.

Will taking ERT help you with your weight? The bottom line is YES, it will for the most part, when coupled with watching your diet. It appears that estrogen stimulates receptors in our abdominal (visceral) fat area so that there is less storage of fat in that area in our premenopausal years. When we go through menopause, estrogen is lower and there is a switch from fat storage in the subcutaneous tissue to the abdominal area. It also appears to that the decline in estrogen in menopause increases activity of the hormone gherlin making us feel less full when we eat so that we eat more. Also estrogen helps us metabolically and appears to have a direct affect on a more favorable lipid profile, causing our "good" HDL cholesterol to be higher.

Central obesity seen in menopause is also commonly found in conditions of higher cortisol (a stress hormone) such as Cushing's disease. It may be that due to the physical and emotional stress of menopause, we produce more cortisol which contributes to fat distribution in our abdomen. Counseling for weight loss recognizes that emotional stress plays a role in weight gain; for example, we crave carbohydrates when tired or will use comfort foods or alcohol as a "reward" for a hard day. Part of the management of menopause will mean adopting practices that help decrease the effects of stress, such as mindfulness and regular breathing exercises.

Several additional factors may contribute to difficulty controlling weight including decreased sleep and changes in mood, which will in turn cause decreased motivation. Some women also have increased joint pain in menopause that makes staying active and exercising a challenge. Also, menopause changes may trigger the onset of Hashimoto's disease resulting in low thyroid hormone levels that directly influence our metabolism and cause weight gain. Women who are experiencing weight gain and fatigue should be checked at least annually for thyroid dysfunction so that this can be addressed and treated appropriately. It is also important to screen for depression, anxiety and insomnia during menopause as part of our approach to menopause treatment strategies. Enlist the support of a dietician and partner who will encourage your long-term goals of a lifetime of healthy eating and regular exercise.

Unfortunately, obesity is an epidemic in many developed countries and women will commonly enter menopause with five to twenty pounds over their ideal weight. Long-term weight studies show that for many adults weight is gained over the winter holidays and never taken off in January. In our society, many of our celebrations center around eating large amounts of fatty or sugary foods. We can easily fall into the trap of family and friends encouraging us to eat more and to drink alcohol when it may not be on our food plan. This results in a slow, gradual weight gain as we age. Address weight issues before menopause so you are starting menopause at an ideal weight with tools for weight maintenance. These tools may include tracking food intake with an easy to use diet app, weighing daily and incorporating exercise into your weekly routine. This can be accomplished with a smart watch and application, or online weight loss or fitness program.

With so many diet plans claiming to be the most effective, which should you choose? In general, the most successful, sustainable diets involve counting carbohydrates and/or calories. For women who have a strong family history of diabetes or have pre-diabetes themselves, start by limiting daily intake of carbohydrates to 125 grams a day. Why? Carbohydrates tend to increase insulin production, which is the body's "storage hormone" for energy and tends to be over secreted in diabetes and metabolic syndromes. Insulin will get very high after a high-carbohydrate meal causing a rapid decline of blood sugar resulting in a "sugar crash" or feeling very tired and hungry within hours of eating. This will result in swings of energy throughout the day due to a cycle of very high and low blood sugars. Focus instead on high-protein meals that include fiber, such as in whole grains and vegetables.

The role of exercise alone in contributing to weight loss has been poor, specifically when diet modifications are not made simultaneously. Paradoxically, it appears that exercise increases appetite and may result in eating more calories than were lost during the exercise cycle. That said, exercise can promote weight maintenance long-term and does help with stress reduction, which can also help long term weight loss. In other words, there is not good evidence that just increasing the number of days you exercise will help you lose weight without also including watching your food intake; however, exercise will help you maintain a healthy weight. In addition, exercise is very important for maintaining a healthy heart and prevent dementia as you age and should be continued for a healthy lifestyle.

Testosterone and weight

One of the hormones that also decreases for women in menopause is testosterone. This hormone has widely been studied for its effects on muscle mass and performance for male athletes. It appears to have a direct effect on our lean muscle mass. Therefore, when women go through menopause, their lean muscle mass decreases, especially if they are not concentrating on weight bearing exercise. Having higher levels of lean muscle results in an increased basal metabolic rate—this is how many calories your body needs each day during rest times. So if you have more lean muscle, your resting metabolic rate will be higher and you will burn through more calories a day at rest. If you have less lean muscle, your body will not require as many calories a day and what you eat in excess of your daily requirement will be stored as fat. Lean muscle can be increased or maintained with weight bearing exercise done at least three times a week. Not only will it help your muscles and keep your metabolism higher, it will increase your bone density and help prevent fractures during aging. Testosterone therapy may be considered as it will also increase lean muscle mass. We will talk further about the complications and benefits of testosterone therapy for women in chapter seven.

Even for scientists, the interactions of these metabolic changes during menopause are not well understood, and much more research needs to be done. Keep informed of diet recommendations that have scientifically backed research from credible sources, and when unsure, talk to your healthcare provider about what is best for you. In summary, maintaining weight involves finding a holistic balance including a nutritious, whole-food diet rich in vegetables and whole grains with high-quality proteins such as fish, eggs and meat. Keep active with aerobic exercise five days a week and manage stress. Consider hormone therapy in this balance for weight loss as well. Remember, since your medical health changes each year, it is most helpful to have a provider who can address issues as they come up year after year and help you decide if ERT is still right for you in finding this healthy balance.

Chapter Five:
Vaginal Care and Sex

Cher
I do think that when it comes to aging, we're held to a different standard than men. Some guy said to me: 'Don't you think you're too old to sing rock n' roll?' I said: 'You'd better check with Mick Jagger'." — *Fifty on Fifty: Wisdom, Inspiration, and Reflections on Women's Lives Well Lived* **by Bonnie Miller Rubin, November 1998**

Let's talk about that beautiful, uniquely feminine organ—the vagina. What amazing resilience it has: it changes with our hormones throughout our lifetimes, responding to signals to become more stretchy for childbirth, and more moist to help the sperm reach the egg, promoting fertility. Unfortunately, when we get to that phase in life when our bodies are no longer able to have children, those vagina-enriching hormones, testosterone, progesterone, and estrogen, are no longer being made. This results in vaginal lining thinning (also called vaginal atrophy), less mucous and fluid being produced, and decreased ability of the vagina to stretch. Much as the skin on our arms and legs thins and is more prone to tearing as we age, the vaginal lining also thins, resulting in painful small and large tears that may bleed during intercourse. In addition, this repetitive association with pain and intercourse may also result in involuntary spasm of the muscles around the vagina when penetration is attempted, worsening the pain of intercourse.

The symptoms of vaginal dryness and pain with intercourse are unique symptoms of menopause since they tend to get worse after menopause—sometimes starting 10-15 years after a woman's last period. Often, I will consult with women who did very well through menopause, with few hot flashes, discovering years later that they have developed severe vaginal dryness in their 60s that won't respond to over-the-counter lubricants. Worsening of this symptom can be a normal progression years after menopause. Combined with decreased libido due to lower testosterone, this pain with intercourse is a condition that decreases the motivation to have sex as we age.

There are other changes that are occurring in other organs of our pelvis as we age, including the bladder and ovaries. Decreased estrogen also ages the bladder and results in increased incidence of urinary tract infection, incontinence, and frequency of urination symptoms. The uterus and ovaries will shrink as we age and the ligaments that supports our bladder and uterus become stretched due to childbirth and/or gravity. Over time this may result in uterine, bladder and rectal prolapse out the vaginal opening. For some women this will need to be fixed with surgery to remove the uterus and tighten the pelvic floor. However, for most women pelvic floor and bladder pain and dysfunction can be treated with physical therapy and vaginal estrogen as we will discuss. Because of the mentioned cascade of events that can happen to the pelvic organs and vagina as we age, being proactive and seeking care from a good provider early can result in better outcomes long term and more interest in a healthy sex life.

Using vaginal estrogens can have many benefits and may be considered as a woman's only estrogen therapy. Topical vaginal estrogens help reverse those changes of vaginal thinning and shortening in a few short weeks, resulting very quickly in pleasurable intercourse and fewer urinary symptoms. Also, it takes very low doses of estrogen to accomplish this—usually 0.1 mg of estradiol taken vaginally twice a week for maintenance verses 1.0mg of estradiol daily taken orally. Because it is a cream, a woman can decide for herself the minimal dose needed to help control symptoms of dryness, sometimes as little as half a gram inserted with an applicator two to three times a week. Also, it can be stopped without causing hot flashes since it is a much lower dose compared to oral estrogen tablets which need to be tapered to avoid hot flashes. It is so effective for helping the vagina and pelvic tissues that some gynecological surgeons will recommend using estrogen for two weeks to a month prior to surgery to help the tissues heal faster after surgery by improving blood flow to the mucosal tissues of the vagina.

Presented here are some of the options for vaginal dryness and atrophy. Keep in mind that they are much lower doses of estrogen in these preparations than are found in other estrogen therapies for hot flashes or bone promotion. For a tailored approach to HRT, they can also be added to other HRT regimens for additional help with vaginal dryness or bladder issues or used as singular therapy for a woman's entire lifetime. In higher dose preparations, the vagina also will absorb this estrogen and release it to body, providing some systemic treatment as well. Because of the vagina's reliable ability to absorb hormones, complete hormone therapy can be given vaginally as a cream, suppository, tablet or ring to help with symptoms of menopause, such as hot flashes.

The hormonal options for topical vaginal treatment are also listed again on the reference chart in Chapter Nine on Hormonal Therapy options for menopause.

Estradiol cream - This is the most prescribed form of vaginal estrogen. A common brand name is Estrace and it is provided in a tube with and applicator that the patient fills to desired dose, usually 1/2 or 1 gram. It is inserted vaginally at bedtime. Patients may use a pea size dollop on the outside near the urethra as well (the opening to the bladder). For severe dryness or vaginal atrophy, patients will use 1/2-1 gram every night for two weeks and then go down to three times a week or less. As mentioned before, this can be decreased to one to two times a week based on a women's satisfaction with results.

Conjugated estrogen cream - A common brand name is Premarin cream. It can be administered as mentioned above in the section on estradiol.

Vagifem tablets - These are small tablets with an applicator inserted twice a week and dissolves slowly to help the mucosa. It is preferred by some women since it does not leak out of the vagina like a cream.

Estring - This is a unique delivery system in that it is a pliable, small ring that is inserted vaginally and will provide continuous estrogen over a three-month period of time. It can be expensive, but remember each ring is about three months of treatment when considering cost.

Estriol 1-4 mg/ gram compounded cream - This is not a standard prescription but is made at a compounded pharmacy. This E3 form of estrogen is very effective for treating vaginal dryness WITHOUT the potential rick of clot formation or stimulation of breast cancer.

Osphena 60 mg pill - This is taken orally once a day. It is an estrogen agonist/antagonist that may have side effects similar to estrogen in that it can increase risk of endometrial or uterine cancer. It also can increased blood clots. It appears to target vaginal tissue and will help significantly in alleviating dryness.

Uva Ursi - An herbal that can promote lubrication of the vagina and healthy bladder function.

Progesterone cream - A compounded cream that can be taken topically on the inner thigh and inner arms can help bladder and vaginal dryness in estrogen-naive patients.

Laser treatments - This includes the Mona Lisa laser in which laser light is used in the vaginal/perineal area to help rejuvenate the tissues and promote small blood vessels and collagen formation. It can be useful for women who cannot take estrogen due to blood clots or breast cancer history. Treatments take five to 15 minutes and are usually every six weeks for about four to six sessions.

As I mentioned earlier, there is a cascade of vaginal thinning, ligament laxity and muscle spasms in response to the pain in the vaginal area, which all contribute to symptoms of dryness or pain with intercourse. Once the vaginal thinning and dryness is addressed, some women still suffer with pain during intercourse. At that point, they may consider a referral to a physical therapist trained in pelvic floor rehabilitation. What can be learned during pelvic floor physical therapy may be life-altering for patients as it can help with urinary symptoms/incontinence and help with mild forms of bladder and uterine prolapse. It can also help treatment for painful vaginismus or pelvic muscle spasming that may be developing. Keep in mind that there are many wonderful, experienced physical therapists nationwide who specialize in pelvic floor rehabilitation. You may consider this in your treatment regime during your discussion with your provider. If a woman continues to have pain with intercourse, their provider may screen for other causes of pelvic pain. This may include evaluation for low back issue and nerve-related pain or ultrasound evaluation for pelvic masses, as examples.

For treatment of vaginal, bladder and uterine prolapse, some women may consider the use of a pessary as they age. Pessaries are devices to support the pelvic floor. They are inserted by a provider into the vagina (much like a diaphragm contraceptive) and "fitted" to your internal pelvis anatomy depending on what size and shape is needed. Pessaries come in many sizes and shapes and work by providing support to the bladder, uterus and rectum during activity. You must find a provider that can help with proper fitting—usually a gynecologist or primary care physician. For some women these are a last resort prior to surgery for repair of a bladder or uterine prolapse; however, they can be very useful for mild cases as well.

As women become more aware of the capacity for better vaginal function and active sex life after menopause, more treatments will most likely become available. Therefore, it is in your best interest to be vocal about your concerns and desires to your healthcare provider. Of course there are some women who may choose another path, perhaps because they have a partner who is also loosing interest or has a medical condition that makes intercourse impossible. You create your romantic relationship based on what is best for you and your partner. Remember, if you desire more enjoyable vaginal sex in your relationship, it may be attainable.

Libido and Testosterone

Libido in all women is a very complex topic—in addition to having a possible biological origin there is a definite psychological component involving our desires and imagination as well as stress levels during our life at the time, such as child rearing and work stress. Because the origin of decreased libido is complex, involving mental and physical processes, it is hard to treat. Biologically, there is a decrease in testosterone in women post-menopausal due to ovarian function decline, often declining at the same time as estrogen. This can happen in the premenopausal or postmenopausal periods. The hormone testosterone is a major player in libido for both men and women. In addition to helping libido, testosterone can help energy and build more lean muscle in women as well contribute to better strength and toning.

Testosterone levels are further jeopardized by estrogen treatments. Women who are on estrogen therapy alone may experience a decrease of free testosterone while on therapy. This is due to stimulation of a protein, sex hormone binding globulin, which may bind testosterone and make it less available in our bloodstream. Fortunately, we can test for total and free testosterone as well as sex hormone binding globulin (SHBG) and identify each patient's status with this hormone to determine if supplementation is needed.

How do we replace it? There is only one standard or pharmaceutical form of FDA-approved prescription testosterone for women in the United States that can be prescribed called Estratest or Estratest HS. This is a tablet form of hormone therapy taken orally that has estradiol and testosterone at low doses, and may help libido somewhat. What is interesting about this option is that testosterone is not well absorbed when taken orally, so its effectiveness is decreased in pill form.

Fortunately, there are several compounded options for women that are better absorbed: testosterone gel used topically or testosterone pellets that are compounded and inserted under the skin every month. Compounded prescriptions must be made at an independent compounding pharmacy or by a pharmacist trained in making pharmaceuticals. These can be made in doses based on a patient's baseline testosterone level and symptoms. In my practice, patients report that topical testosterone helps improve libido or desire for increased sex about 65 percent of the time. Since it is topical, the dose can be adjusted by applying more or less gel or using it more or fewer days of the week. A typical dose is two to six milligrams applied topically to thin skin on the body (usually on the back of the arms or inner thighs). Recently, an application to the FDA for a testosterone patch for women was evaluated and declined. It has some good data in Europe for helping with libido in post-menopausal women and hopefully an alternative will be available soon. Testosterone has several potential side effects for women: increasing acne (even if you are older), increasing facial hair, and deepening a woman's voice. Larger doses of testosterone may also make a woman feel aggressive and can increase insomnia.

As mentioned before, there is also an emotional component to decreased libido. For many women, the setting and foreplay surrounding a sexual encounter is very important to promoting interest in sexual activity. Create time when you are not feeling overextended and tired for intimacy with your partner. As we will discuss in Chapter eight, menopause affects your mood and may result in increased depression, anxiety, and mental fogginess that may leave you feeling overwhelmed and tired. Make time for self-love and relaxation. You deserve it and it will influence your desire for sex in the long term.

Remember that there are usually two people involved in having a satisfying sex-life. Talk to your partner about your concerns, symptoms and desires. Overcoming these mental roadblocks are very important for most women to help with increased sexual desire. A couple may consider professional help with a counselor if needed. Chances are your partner will be very interested in learning more; women's changes during menopause are as mysterious for your partner as they are for you! Let your partner be involved and get creative; there may be more your partner can do to satisfy you if you are open to communicating your dislikes and desires.

Chapter Six:
Menopause and Your Bones

As we have reviewed earlier, menopause is a time for physical changes that may vary depending on the individual; however, there is one change that affects all women after cessation of periods, and that is a gradual decrease in bone density making the bones prone to spontaneous fractures as a woman ages. Since it affects all women to different degrees based on lifestyle and genetics, it may influence a woman's choice of whether to start a hormonal estrogen versus non-hormonal management of menopause. Estrogen therapy has been proven time and time again to preserve bones after menopause in study after study. Starting an estrogen therapy option at the beginning of menopause seems to stop the usual decrease of bone density found in the first ten years after menopause. The timing of initiation of estrogen therapy is crucial, as estrogen must be started just after menopause begins in order to help maintain bone density. In other words, if you started menopause at 50, you cannot decide to take estrogen at 65 to help your bones. Apparently, there is a window of five years after menopause when the addition of estrogen is most beneficial. As we shall discuss, there are several other medications that may be used for women who cannot take estrogen or have missed that window. There are also important lifestyle changes that can help bone density that all women should start in their 40-50s if they haven't already by that time.

Most women do not realize that they have lower bone density or are at risk for fractures in their spine and hip as they age. Women with osteoporosis (severe low bone density) often do not realize that they have decreased bone density since there are no apparent symptoms early on and screening is recommended later in life, usually age 65. Because of this delay, one may not recognize this disorder until it manifests as a spontaneous fracture of the spine or hip. In the early stages, osteoporosis does not cause pain or deformity. This is why having a discussion with your provider about screening for osteoporosis at the beginning of menopause is important. Screening for bone density is usually done with a DEXA or bone density scan, which measures the concentration of the bone in the hip and lumbar spine and often the wrist. It is a quick, painless procedure that is recommended every five to six years when screening for osteoporosis. According to the United States Preventative Task Force (USPTF), all women should be screened at 65 years of age, however, this would be well past the age of starting estrogen for menopause, which on average starts at age 50.

There are some women who are more at risk for developing osteoporosis. If you have low body weight or are a smoker, you are more at risk. If you have a family history in your mother or older sibling of osteoporosis or hip and spine fracture you are at increased risk. Keep in mind that for older generations, a DEXA scan may not have been available—if you remember having relatives with a kyphotic hump or hunchback, they may have had osteoporosis and had not been aware of spontaneous fractures occuring their spine. Other medical conditions that may increase risk are thyroid disease, long-term steroid use for autoimmune issues or asthma, celiacs disease and inflammatory bowel disease. Also low estrogen states like early menopause or a complete hysterectomy at an early age, lack of periods from anorexia, or being an extreme athlete may increase your risk. If you have one of these increased risk factors, you may consider getting a DEXA scan at menopause or earlier to determine if estrogen may be beneficial to preserving your bones. There is an online tool called the FRAX assessment that will help to calculate your risk for spontaneous fracture based on your age, weight and risk factors.

Bone density or DEXA scan results are a bit unusual as the number that is calculated is a negative number. This is because it is a ratio of an average woman's bone density at age 20 or 30 (usually peak bone density age) with the woman being tested who is usually over 50 years old. DEXA results have several data points reported. It will show a T-score and a Z-score as well as a percent decrease from previous scans if done. Results also include a patient-specific ten-year risk of having a spontaneous fracture. For simplicity it is best to look at the T-score in determining if a woman falls into normal, osteopenia or osteoporosis categories. Here is the usual breakdown: T-score value of less than -1.0 is normal, between -1.0 and -2.5 is osteopenia and less than -2.5 is osteoporosis. In general, it is very challenging, even with medications and extreme lifestyle changes to increase bone density after menopause. However, many medications will stabilize bone and prevent progression to fractures despite the lack of increased bone density.

As I mentioned before, our overall health plays a part in preserving bone density, and there are healthy lifestyle choices that can be made to help improve bone density. Avoiding cigarettes and caffeine may be helpful. A diet rich in calcium can help (600-1200 mg a day), or if you are not obtaining this amount daily in your diet, the addition of a calcium supplement may be needed. This is especially important in our 20s and 30s when we are building our peak bone mass. Vitamin D helps the colon to absorb calcium from the gut and is therefore important in bone health. Many providers take extra care to ensure that women in menopause have adequate Vitamin D levels by checking blood levels and recommending supplementation if needed. Some practitioners recommend the addition of Vitamin K for absorption, however this has not been well proven to have an impact on bone density.

Weight-bearing exercise is extremely important in preserving bones—at least 30 minutes three times a week involving the upper body and core. This can also be achieved by walking with arm weights or a loaded back pack to increase the load on their hips and spine and increase bone density. If you have the resources, investing in two- to ten-pound weights can be very helpful to maintaining this routine.

There are several medications that may help a woman who has not decided to take estrogen therapy and may have had their first fracture or newly diagnosed osteoporosis. These medications are prescribed if there is a severe progression of bone loss as noted in serial bone density or DEXA scans or when a woman enters the stage of osteoporosis. The goal of treatment is to stop the loss of bone density and to stabilize the bones to avoid spontaneous fracture. The most commonly used are the bisphosphonate class, also knows as Fosamax (the generic name is alendronate sodium) which is taken orally once a week and Boniva (ibandronate) taken once a month. Usually these medications can be taken for five to six years and will work for many years after stopping since they remain in the bones. Also, these medications are often also used for prevention of osteoporosis in women who are at risk due to family history or for first-time treatment of osteoporosis. Side effects of these medications include GERD or heartburn, spontaneous fracture of the femur (although very rare) and osteonecrosis (softening) of the jaw. In our community, many oral surgeons will avoid surgery in patients on bisphosphonates due to this risk involving the jaw and potential for delayed healing. These medications also need to be taken on an empty stomach with a full glass of water, and you must stay upright for 30 minutes after taking to avoid irritation to the esophagus.

Another option for prevention of bone loss is the medication Evista (raloxifene), which is taken once a day; however, this benefits only the spine for improving density. It works as an estrogen receptor mimic and there is some evidence that it may protect against breast cancer. It may increase hot flashes and cause leg cramps. It does not have good evidence in studies for prevention of hip fractures. Therefore, if you have a low T-score of less than -2.5 in your hip indicating osteoporosis, this may not be a good option for you.

For women with osteoporosis or who have failed the bisphosphonates, options include Reclast (zoledronic acid), an infusion done once a year. This is a very good medication for improving bone density, even in the first year of taking it; however, it must be administered in a doctor's office or an infusion center. Most common potential side effects include dizziness, changes in electrolytes and body aches similar to the flu.

Forteo (teriparatide) and Tymlos (abaloparatide), both mimic parathyroid hormone, and are injections done every day for two years; then, patients are put back on a bisphosphenates. Prolia (densumab) is an injection done every six months and slows the progression of bone loss. This is usually administered in a doctor's office but it may be done at home. It may cause skin rashes and inhibit the immune system.

When all else fails, some women will use Miacalcin (calcitonin) nasal spray; however, this is not as effective in maintaining bones and does not have good scientific data proving prevention of fractures in older women. The most common side effects are nasal dryness or nose bleeds and fatigue.

Treating osteoporosis can be done with medications, but it is better to prevent it from occurring as you age. This can be accomplished with hormonal treatments in menopause and certain lifestyle changes in many instances. For some women, it is unavoidable. Remember, that many of the usual treatments for osteoporosis have side effects and are very expensive. With this in mind, considering your bone health as early as you enter menopause is the best strategy so that it weighs into your decision whether to take estrogen therapy. Again, osteoporosis is difficult to diagnose since initially there are no symptoms. Studies show that people who have hip fractures when they are older, say in their 80s, are much more likely to need nursing home care. Taking care of your bones now is insurance for better quality of life when you are older.

Chapter Seven:
Thyroid Issues in Menopause

In the past five to ten years there has been a surge in the use of the internet by patients wanting to gain information about healthcare and find potential diagnoses that may explain a constellation of symptoms that are concerning them. Even among healthcare providers, the use of the internet for relevant health care information is about 90 percent. It is an excellent resource for travel and financial advice and a great place to find a YouTube video on how to patch your wall. However, there is a lot of information that is very inaccurate and misleading, especially when it come to healthcare advice on treatment and diagnosis. Internet searches on each healthcare topic will turn up many anecdotal stories that are heartfelt and compelling but not scientifically valid.

One common diagnosis that patients of any age are sure to make after consulting "Dr. Internet" is thyroid dysfunction or low thyroid. It is understandable why: the most common symptoms of hypothyroid are fatigue and weight gain—nearly all of us have had this in our lives at some point. Often, women will seek medical care in menopause concerned that their thyroid is underfunctioning, stating they have all the symptoms listed in an internet search. What is interesting is that these are the same symptoms of menopause—if you look at the following list you can immediately see the confusion.

Menopause symptoms	**Hypothyroid symptoms**
weight gain centrally	weight gain
fatigue	fatigue
heat intolerance and hot flashes	cold intolerance
sleep disturbance	sleep disturbances or excessive sleep
mental fogginess	mental fogginess
menstrual changes	heavy period or infertility
hair loss	hair loss
dry skin	dry skin
depression or anxiety	depression or anxiety
joint pain	joint pain

As you can clearly see, there are very similar symptoms in both, almost completely overlapping lists. So how can we tell these conditions apart? Luckily, there are blood tests for determining a woman's thyroid level currently. We can measure directly the thyroid hormones and determine from these if there is an issue with under, or over-active thyroid. Women who have a strong family history of thyroid disease are more likely to develop it themselves and should be tested. Thyroid disease is likely to go unrecognized during menopause because the symptoms are so similar and can be explained as due to menopause. To further complicate this issue, menopause may actually contribute to acceleration or activation of thyroid disorders during menopause.

As mentioned before, there are some autoimmune diseases that will become stimulated in women when they are going through menopause—rheumatoid arthritis and lupus for example. Another less commonly known disease is Hashimoto's thyroiditis, a disease in which one's body makes antibodies to one's thyroid and causes inflammation. This may result in periods of time when your thyroid is overactive and times when the thyroid is underactive, cycling between fatigue and overstimulation for many years. Many people with Hashimoto's thyroiditis may look like they have bipolar disease—they have periods of being very stimulated and energetic and times when they are very tired and unmotivated.

To complicate this issue further, the typical blood test we use for screening for thyroid disease may appear normal when a patient has Hashimoto's thyroiditis. This is because there must be very specific lab testing—that is, the thyroid peroxisomal antibodies or TPOAb and, to a lesser extent, anti-thyroglobulin antibodies (TGAb)- that needs to be performed on blood to determine if this disease is active. Unfortunately, traditional medicine does not provide treatment for this condition, and this may be why many physicians do not test for it. However, in a functional or naturopathic medicine paradigm, we can provide advice regarding diet and alternative medical options such as herbals that may be helpful once the condition is recognized.

What exactly does your thyroid do? It is a gland located at the bottom of the neck, just above the clavicles and it releases a hormone, thyroxine, that controls metabolism. Metabolism is the process of making energy for your cells to function and affects every system in your body—digestion, brain, weight and body temperature. When a person is experiencing hyperthyroid symptoms and is overactive metabolically, they will feel hot, irritable, have increased appetite with weight loss, diarrhea, rapid heart rate and sometimes hair loss and oily skin. For hypothyroid symptoms it is the opposite: metabolism is decreased and one experiences weight gain, fatigue, constipation, they feel cold all the time and may have dry skin.

If there is so much overlap of symptoms between menopause and thyroid issues, and the menopause can trigger thyroid dysfunction, then how do we determine what is truly going on for a woman? This is where we rely on information from blood testing. For care of my patients, I recommend extensive thyroid testing annually throughout menopause, since symptoms alone are unreliable. The testing is confusing for a person without medical training to interpret: the following explains what is usually included in a thyroid panel of blood tests.

- **Thyroid Stimulating Hormone** (TSH) - This is the only test that most physicians will order for initial thyroid evaluation, so it is commonly reported. The normal range is typically between 0.35 m/L and 3.5 m/L. The value measured is actually the hormone that is made by your pituitary gland in your brain to help stimulate your thyroid. So if it is low then your thyroid is **overproducing** thyroid hormone and if it is high then you thyroid is **underproducing** thyroid hormone. Read this carefully because this is completely different than what you would expect looking at the results. To complicate interpretation further, the results of normal vary according to the lab. Usually a value above 4.0 is a high TSH signal from the pituitary gland meaning that thyroid hormone is low in the blood-stream and diagnostic for hypothyroidism or low thyroid. However, not everyone with low thyroid needs to be treated right away with medications. If the TSH is between 4-13 m/L and one does not have symptoms, thyroid medication may not be needed. In fact, for many years, a TSH value below 5.5 and above 0.35 was considered normal. Some patients present with very high TSH levels when first diagnosed with hypothyroid and this value may even be as high as 150 m/L or more. At that level thyroid hormone supplementation is needed.

- **Free T4** - This is the actual measurement of hormones made by your thyroid gland. The word "free" refers to the amount that is not bound by proteins in the blood and available to the cells. It is based on a range for the general population across many age ranges and weights, which may explain why some people have normal thyroid but slightly abnormal Free T4 levels. Most medications for thyroid are thyroxine (T4).

- **Free T3** - This is the hormone that is made at the cellular level; T4 is converted into T3 at the cellular level and this is its active form, which will result in increased metabolism at the cellular level. Some people have a decreased ability to make this conversion and this needs to be replaced specifically in medication form as T3.

- **Thyroid Antibodies** - Thyroid peroxisomal antibodies (TPO) and antithyroglobulin antibodies. These can be high in Hashimoto's thyroiditis and Grave's disease—both autoimmune thyroid disorders.

Most cases of hypothyroidism during menopause are because of damage to the thyroid from Hashimoto's thyroiditis. As mentioned before, it can cause enlargement and tenderness of the thyroid gland and symptoms of low and high thyroid, but this process may also occur without symptoms at all. This type of thyroiditis can cause a long, slow progressive burnout of thyroid over years, or it can happen in an aggressive phase over a few months. For either type, the thyroid eventually burns out completely and will stop making thyroid hormone.

Graves' disease is another autoimmune thyroid condition in which people make antibodies to the receptor on the thyroid, which directly stimulates the thyroid. For most, this results in a very enlarged thyroid that is tender, and it may be difficult to swallow due to the thyroid's location. It also causes hyperthyroidism with racing heart, weight loss, diarrhea and trouble sleeping. The treatment is generally more aggressive for this and consultation with an endocrinologist is required.

There is not a lot of good scientific data on how to approach Hashimoto's thyroiditis in traditional medicine. This is unfortunate since recognition and treatment using a functional medicine approach may help stabilize an individual's physical and mental state as well as slow the progression to daily requirement of thyroid hormone. This requires aggressive diet intervention and addition of supplements to help heal the gut. This approach can be useful for other types of autoimmune disease that may present in menopause. In functional/alternative medicine, the "leaky gut syndrome" model explains why we focus on the digestive track and diet when we are dealing with a hormonal issue.

Leaky gut syndrome is a theory that provides a possible explanation for why changes in diet and attention to our microbiome seems to help people feel better, even improving autoimmune diseases for some people. Basically the theory states that over time our gut becomes more permeable, exposing our blood stream to food and bacteria in our gut. It is uncertain why this happens, but may be related to food allergies, antibiotics that we take and environmental toxins like pesticides in our foods. Because of this increased "leakiness" in our gut, we start to have an exaggerated immune response and produce more antibodies to our foods. So as we eat even healthy foods, we produce an immune response, increasing inflammation in the intestines. Our bodies recognize food falsely as an invader and will increase cytokines, prostaglandins, antibodies and some hormones like cortisol to "fight" the invader. As a results, patients feel chronically sick and may have increased stomach bloating, diarrhea and gassiness when eating foods. Some people go many years feeling bad, mounting this response slowly over time. Changes in our immune system during menopause increase this response with exaggerated T-cell and interferon production, the same chemicals released during inflammation.

The diet advice that follows is based on functional medicine studies and experience with patients. Changing your diet can be challenging, so we have chosen what is simplest and most effective for the majority of patients based on improvement on thyroid testing, sometimes without the need for medications. To make it simple, we combine supplements with dietary restrictions initially as follows:

- First, start eating an organic diet with fewer processed foods—this will eliminate unnecessary antibiotics, hormones and preservatives.

- Try to avoid or limit alcohol, as it has a profound affect on liver function and seems to decrease intestinal mucous production.

- Add a broad spectrum, high potency probiotic to your daily routine.

- Eliminate gluten and wheat entirely from your diet. Bread, pasta and wheat appear to be very allergenic for a lot of individuals who have had negative celiac testing; this may be because of how it is processed. Many patients may see a lowering of TPO antibodies after a few months of a gluten-free diet for those with Hashimoto's thyroiditis.

- Consider eliminating other common foods that cause allergies such as soy, dairy, nuts, corn, and eggs. Just try one at a time for two weeks and see how you feel. Do you have more energy and better bowel function? Chances are you have an allergy to that food and it should be avoided.

- Add glutamine powder or pills as a supplement prior to meals to decrease gut inflammation.

- Add Aloe Vera juice as well to soothe the intestinal lining and help with inflammation.

Once a patient has tried these interventions for a few months, we recommend checking blood work including a thyroid panel and see if there is improvement in symptoms. For patients with a positive response in symptoms and labs, we recommend continuing these modifications for two years and then consider adding foods in gradually. For people who do not respond, we may consider doing specific food allergy testing and a comprehensive stool analysis (CDSA) for more detailed approach. A CDSA testing kit can be obtained by participating providers and will measure stool for bacteria content (both beneficial and harmful), parasites, yeast, fungus, products of digestion that may be lacking including enzymes, pH and inflammatory cells.

What has been outlined regarding healing the intestines and decreasing inflammation in this chapter is not common knowledge among traditionally trained physicians. In order to accomplish your goals, you may need to work with a physician trained in functional medicine or a reputable naturopathic physician. However, interventions provided do not require a prescription and can be done on your own if you are very suspicious of having a dysfunctional thyroid.

Chapter Eight:
Menopause and Your Brain

Toni Morrison
"At 81, I don't feel guilty about anything ... There's nothing inside that's 81. It's just the changes in the body. And the memory. I don't remember where the keys are. Or as my son says, 'Ma, it's not that you don't remember where you put the keys, it's when you pick up your keys and you don't know what they're for'." — *The Guardian*, April 2012

In the past five years there has been an increase in study of the human brain driven in part by a desire for treatment options for those stricken by disabling diseases including Alzheimer's disease, multiple sclerosis and other neurodegenerative disease. We have also seen increased study on the impact of hormonal decline on our blood vessels and nervous system both which affect our brain functioning. There are new frontiers of study on the intersection of aging and lifestyle, the role of epigenetics in aging, and the influences of our environment on our biological processes. With each new revelation come complexities in how this information may apply to each and every one of us on a practical level, especially when it comes to our brains and the risk of progression to dementia, stroke or Alzheimer's disease. In this section we will focus on recent discoveries of how the hormonal changes of menopause effect the brain.

Some of you may already have experienced that menopause brought with it extreme changes in your cognitive function. Many women that I see in my practice complain of "brain fog" or not being able to multi-task as they used to. As a practicing physician, for years I was perplexed as to why this was such a common complaint around menopause, occurring in women almost as much as hot flashes. Was this decline in brain functioning related to lack of sleep from frequent hot flashes? Or was the onset of depression due to the challenges of aging? Coincidentally, I found that treating menopausal women with estrogen early on helped sleep and hot flashes and seemed to improve some of that mental sharpness that had been lost. A more likely explanation is on the horizon: we are coming to a clearer understanding of what is happening to the brain during menopause, and there is increasing evidence that cognitive function can be improved with hormonal and other interventions.

Recent scientific findings show there are significant changes happening in the brain during menopause, specifically measurable inflammation. According to Wang et al., 2020, from the University of Arizona, as we age there is a change in our brain metabolism from primarily glucose metabolism to fatty acid and ketone metabolism, which is a switch from a quick source of energy to a more complex form of energy for the brain. In addition there is direct damage to cellular structures in the brain, increasing free radical formation and a cascade of inflammatory markers in the brain. This translates to measurable inflammation and damage to neurons and surrounding blood vessels in the perimenopausal to menopausal transition, a change that can be seen microscopically in the brains of mice who are forced into menopause. As we get years past our transition, our brains adapt to these metabolic and hormonal changes and inflammation lessens.

They authors go on to explain that estrogen can decrease these changes and help cognitive function if given within five years of starting menopause. Studies done on menopausal rats showed microscopic improvement of inflammation in brain structures when they were given estrogen. In other words, taking estrogen just before and during the first few years of menopause has a protective effect on your brain against developing Alzheimer's and provides a clarifying effect on cognitive function immediately. This is remarkably compelling piece of evidence supporting estrogen therapy for many women, especially if you have a strong family history of Alzheimer's disease or have a genetic marker, such as APOE4 that increases your risk for Alzheimer's disease.

There are also other metabolic changes happening in our bodies that may contribute to damage to the small blood vessels in our brains. Weight gain as well as epigenetic expression of inherited genes from our parents may result in the start of high blood pressure, high cholesterol and diabetes. These medical conditions set us up for strokes and small-vessel disease in the brain that may be irreversible. A comprehensive approach to keeping our brains functioning well after menopause must include screening for these diseases with regular physical exams and blood tests to make sure that you are not developing one of these conditions. .

Keep in mind that even if you develop diabetes, hypertension or high cholesterol in the post-menopausal period, your first line of treatment will be to modify your lifestyle: stop smoking, increase your exercise and watch your diet. Let me say that again another way; if you do the hard work of counting your carbohydrates, eating an organic diet of unprocessed foods and exercising daily, you can prevent long-term brain atrophy, Alzheimer's dementia and avoid a stroke as you age. It cannot be emphasized enough that a heathy lifestyle as you age is not just about looking thin or younger; it is about good mental functioning (as well as protection against heart disease and cancer).

Speaking of a healthy diet for the brain, there are several other points to emphasize about eating as we age. Since your brain metabolism is switching to using fats as its food source as you age, it is important that your diet is rich in good fats such as essentially fatty acids and omega-3 and omega-6 fatty acids. Examples of beneficial fats include olive oils, chia seeds, flax seed oil, avocados, cold water fish and coconut oil. Also, a vitamin B12 supplement should be added daily since we loose our ability to absorb this vitamin in our intestines. In fact, B12 deficiency may start with symptoms of neuropathy, or numbness in feet, and dementia as we age. In addition, vitamin B12 deficiency is more prevalent in people who drink alcohol regularly. There is also evidence that correcting vitamin D deficiency may protect against Alzheimer's disease. Also, a diet low in carbohydrates decreases our circulating levels of insulin, a hormone we make when we eat which may also contribute to vascular disease and neurogenic toxicity.

Some studies show benefits to our brains when we regularly schedule times of intermittent fasting, since it stimulates a hormone called brain derived growth factor (abbreviated BDGF) which is beneficial for neurogenesis and concentration. This is accomplished by not eating food for 12-48 hour periods of time once or twice a week. Typically you can have clear liquids during that time. One example of this strategy would be to not eat snacks after your evening meal at 6 pm and to eat again at lunch time at noon the next day. This would be the equivalent of an 18-hour fast.

Protect your brain health at all costs—it is THE most important factor to enjoying life as we age. You have earned years of wisdom by the time you reach menopause, now is the time to articulate your wisdom and lead the next generation.

Keeping your brain healthy is not just about stopping progression to devastating disease as we age. It is also about living our best life in this next phase. Many women work years by the time they are in menopause and are really reaching their optimum abilities in their careers, climbing the executive ladder or becoming tenured at a university. Now is the time for us to shine and be leaders so that we can influence our world to better the next generation. Or perhaps you have spent many years raising children and finally have time to go back to school, write a book or start a new career—this is YOUR time. The sky is the limit. You need a well-functioning brain to accomplish this. Even if your goal is to relax and focus on self care or travel, you will need good brain functioning to manage retirement and finances. Protect it at all costs.

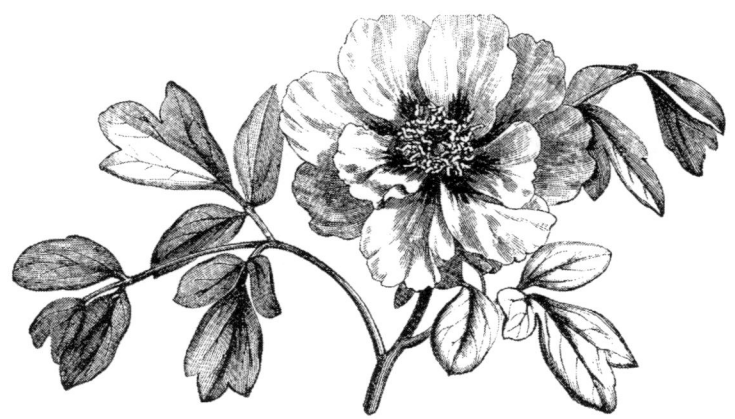

Fig. 3. Flowering Branch of Pæonia Moutan.

Chapter Nine: Hormonal Treatment Approach to Menopause

This comes as a surprise to many patients but currently there is not a consensus among physicians regarding the best hormonal treatment for symptoms of menopause, or if menopause should be treated at all with hormone therapy due to potential risks. Menopause truly is a natural, normal process and there are a large number of women who stop having periods and have few symptoms, such as hot flashes. After careful consideration of the risks and benefits, many women may decide to do without additional treatments and allow menopause to progress naturally. Sometimes women will choose to start hormones for reasons such as protection of bones or preservation of vaginal health. On the other hand, if a woman has a mother who had breast cancer at an early age, they may decide to avoid estrogen therapies to decrease the possibility of stimulating breast cancer later in life. The decision of whether hormone therapy should be started depends on each individual woman's experience of symptoms, goals in treatment, and risks due to family or medical history.

My approach to consultation for a woman seeking options during menopause is very holistic and involves knowledge of their current medical conditions, family history, lifestyle choices and what symptoms they are currently having that are affecting their daily life. Usually we are able to make initial treatment based on this discussion and desired long-term outcome. I may elect to do blood work to confirm that they are truly in menopause and can no longer get pregnant or to check on hormone levels. However, not all women need to have lab testing to get initial treatment. We may also try herbals or acupuncture first based on my patient's comfort level with hormones or one's desire to stay off prescriptions entirely. Typically the process of navigating menopause involves a lot of discussion between my patient and myself as well as some trial and error. As I said before, one size does not fit all.

There is an overwhelming number of options for hormone replacement therapy (HRT) and the length of time for treatment depends on what we are trying to treat or achieve long term for each individual patient. It will also depend on whether the patient has increased risk factors for heart disease or breast cancer in their family or other medical conditions that may be made worse with hormonal treatment. In this section, we will review standard medication options you can obtain with a prescription from your family physician or gynecologist. In the next chapter we will discuss compounded or bio-identical hormones: these are made at a compounding pharmacy only with varying amounts of hormones based on patient/physician preference and goals of treatment. Keep in mind that compounded hormones, bio-identical hormones and natural hormones are terms used interchangeably. Compounded prescriptions are generally not covered by most insurance companies and cost varies by pharmacy.

Once we have determine that hormone replacement therapy is indicated and desired by the patient, lower doses of hormones are initiated and gradually increased based on how well symptoms are being controlled, keeping close attention to unwanted side effects. If a patient seems to be getting to higher prescription doses of estrogen, progesterone or testosterone than expected, blood levels may be checked to make sure that we are not getting too high and placing a patient at risk for complications.

Most physicians do not typically advocate testing regularly to make sure a patient is in a certain range of hormone level in their bodies. There are several reasons for this. First there is no scientific evidence that supports a need for hormones in a certain range for longevity or quality of life. Secondly, with blood, salivary and urine testing there is too much fluctuation throughout the day and week to support a "target" level beyond a range of where hormones should be for an individual. Thirdly, some women (and men) have no symptoms and have very low sex hormone levels. In fact many patients have very normal libido and no hot flashes and have extremely low levels of hormones on testing. Lab testing is for guidance only and should be paired with an in-depth knowledge of the patient and their concerns and goals. Testing can be accomplished by blood, urine or salivary samples.

Standard Prescription Hormonal Options

For a patient who is new to HRT, we will typically start with a standard prescription first: these are hormones you can get at any pharmacy with a doctor's prescription. Standard prescriptions have the advantage of being easier to obtain and less costly since they are generally included on a patient's formulary, meaning prescriptions covered by one's insurance company. Also, if there are negative side effects such as breast tenderness, headaches, or nausea, the doses can be changed easily with another prescription. The easiest and most common form is oral, once-a-day pills; however, there are also patches and vaginal forms of estrogen that may be more appropriate. Please refer to charts at the end of this chapter. Also note charts for compounded hormones, which will be discussed in the next chapter.

Basically there are two forms of estrogen available in standard prescriptions: conjugated estrogens (not to be confused with compounded estrogen, discussed later) and estradiol. Estradiol is the same estrogen that is often in bioidentical estrogens, also called compounded estrogens, but found in combinations with DHEA, progesterone and testosterone when compounded for the individual. Estradiol topically is also supplied as a patch in standard prescriptions, either reapplied once or twice a week. This has the advantage of avoiding issues of absorption by the intestines—either by food intake, intestinal malabsorption issues and interference by other medications taken orally. Topical estrogens have the additional benefit of bypassing "first-pass metabolism." This means that estrogen taken topically circulates through the body before it is broken down by the liver during normal metabolism of the drug. For oral hormones, the medication must first go from the intestines to the liver (where it may be partially metabolized) before it goes to the rest of the body. Injectable estradiol is another potentially convenient form of estrogen since it is injected every three to four weeks; it also bypasses liver metabolism initially, resulting in a larger amounts of the desired hormone in the tissues. There is also vaginal estrogen—both estradiol and conjugated estrogens—which were described in a separate chapter on vaginal health. Vaginal estrogens also bypass the liver and may be used for complete HRT, especially the tablet or vaginal ring forms of estrogen.

Those women who have not had a hysterectomy by the time they are on estrogen therapy should also take progesterone. This is to protect the uterus from stimulation of the endometrial lining by estrogen that can result in endometrial cancer. It appears that only a low dose of progesterone is needed to accomplish this—as little as ten days worth every three months. Progesterone is also supplied in standard prescriptions with estrogen in pills and patch form. Many women prefer micronized progesterone, also known as the brand name Prometrium, a standard prescription in tablet form. It does not appear to have as much bloating or weight gain as can be found with other forms of progesterone—especially medroxyprogesterone. If you have had a hysterectomy, it is not necessary to take progesterone with your HRT since there is not a concern for endometrial cancer.

A preferred standard prescription combination for women is the combination of an estradiol patch changed twice a week with a micronized progesterone tablet every night. Be aware that for some women the adhesive in the patch is irritating to the skin or the patch falls off easily. However, this form of estrogen appears to work well for many symptoms of menopause without side effects. Because there are two prescriptions (and two expected co-pays for insurance purposes), many women will opt for estradiol/norethidrone acetate (progesterone) as a pill once a day. This is a very simple and affordable option for most patients and will work extremely well for most. The downfall to this option is that there are only two dosing sizes—either 0.5 mg or 1.0 mg based on the estrogen component.

Other combinations of HRT and their brand names are supplied in the table at the end of this chapter. My experience is that brand name HRT is very expensive and not covered under most formularies and is not necessarily better at symptom control. You can use this table at the end of this chapter when searching HRT options in your prescription formulary from your insurance company. It is important to consider that non-formulary HRT can cost from $60-$300 a month, making it prohibitive for some patients. Usually, if patients are not getting the benefits they desire from the standard HRT prescriptions, we will suggest compounded (bioidentical) hormones as the next step rather than choose more expensive, brand name standard hormones.

Compounded Hormones

Compounded hormones are prescriptions that are made at a specialized pharmacy for the individual patient with a prescription from a doctor knowledgeable in compounded hormone therapy. These are also commonly referred to by my patients as "natural hormones" or "bioidentical hormones" and erroneously thought of as without the risks of HRT such as stimulation of breast cancer, blood clots or heart attacks. Please note that compounded forms do have estrogens that may still increase your risks associated with standard HRT. Unfortunately, there have not been long-term studies on these formulations to help physicians scientifically assess these risks. There are several aspects of compounded hormones that make them safer: for instance, the amount of estradiol in these preparations is usually much lower than in standard prescriptions (usually just a quarter of the dose). These compounded preparations are made with several types of hormones found naturally in the ovulating female including estriol and estrone—which may help menopause symptoms without the potential risks found in estradiol prescriptions alone. The combination of two or three estrogens is referred to as bi-estrogen or tri-estrogens, respectively, and can be made with progesterone and testosterone as well. Also of benefit is that we can decrease these hormones to the lowest milligram amount that helps control symptoms for that particular patient, resulting in less potential risk to the patient. Compounded hormones have hundreds of dosing options, and they can be made in tablet, sublingual, topical, sub-dermal and vaginal forms, which provides a more tailored approach to the individual patient.

Compounding hormones specific to a patient is complicated and most practitioners will have compounding pharmacists in their area with whom they collaborate. There is an abundance of information specifically from Women's International Pharmacy and often their website will have up-to-date information on the latest research. Some compounding pharmacists can also collaborate with patients and practitioners to provide education and suggestions for an individual patient. As the patient, is important for you to find a team to work with on your path towards wellness during menopause. For most women, I find that initially finding the right dose in your compounded hormone therapy takes some adjustment and testing, once the correct formulation is found, very little adjustment will need to be made in the coming years.

Some providers will recommend compounded pellets that are inserted under the skin once a month and absorbed slowly by the body. These pellets can be made with estrogen, testosterone and progesterone by a compounded pharmacy. Hormones administered this way are convenient since you will not need to take a daily pill prescription. However, it will take time from your schedule to make the appointment to have it inserted. This method also relies on a very skilled compounding pharmacy as small fluctuations in the small batch made by a compounding pharmacist may have unwanted side effects. Once the pellet is inserted, it is not removed. For some this is a preferred option if they do not have side effects. However, women with side effects may experience them over the next month or more, possibly even for years after insertion.

Assessing Risk Factors for Estrogen Replacement Therapy

Every initial conversation regarding management options for menopause should include a discussion of individual risk factors and family history that may influence a woman's decision to take estrogen. There are several contraindications to taking estrogen—these are conditions a woman may have currently that may be worsened or caused by taking estrogen. First, if they have a history of breast cancer, then they should not take estrogen, especially if their cancer is estrogen/progesterone receptor positive as seen on pathology reports. These women are usually also instructed to avoid black cohosh and large amounts of soy containing foods since they are estrogen-like. Even bioidentical or compounded estrogens may be avoided in these women since they may still stimulate cancer growth. It is particularly important that women on hormone therapy get regular mammograms in order to identify cancer at early stages should it develop while on HRT.

We are fortunate at this time to have very good genetic testing to detect some mutations prominent in certain inherited breast cancers. These can be done with blood or saliva in which the DNA in white cells or epithelial cells of these samples is analyzed for certain mutations. Women who have BRACA I or II or Lynch syndrome diagnosed in this manner are at higher risk than the general population—some have a 50 percent increase in breast cancer risk. Those women should not take estrogen therapy. If a woman has a strong family history of breast cancer, ovarian cancer and endometrial cancer, they may think about obtaining genetic testing from their provider prior to initiating therapy. A good resource and pedigree analysis tool for assessing your risk can be found on the Myriad Genetics website. Prior to any genetic testing, it is a good idea to discuss expectations and consequences of having a mutation with a genetics counselor. This service is usually done on-line via telemedicine and may be covered by insurance as well.

Women who smoke cigarettes, even socially, should not take estrogen. Cigarette smoking significantly increases a woman's risk of stroke or heart attacks, which increases exponentially by adding estrogen. Also, please be aware that if you have a personal history of blood clots, either involving the veins or arteries, then you should not consider estrogen therapy. This would include deep vein thrombosis, pulmonary embolism, strokes and heart attacks. The risk of increased clot formation in women is higher on estrogen at any age, including 20 year-old women who take birth control pills. Physicians are particularly careful during evaluation for estrogen therapy in those women who have a higher risk of developing heart attacks or strokes as well. This may mean cardiac testing and evaluation prior to initiating estrogen therapy. That would include if you have an immediate family member (mother or father) with heart disease and strokes; or if you have diabetes, high cholesterol or high blood pressure. There are also some inherited syndromes that predispose women to blood clot formation such as Protein C and S, antithrombin III deficiency, anticardiolipin antibody, and factor V deficiency. Women with primary or secondary polycythemia are also at higher risk for clots.

On the other hand, estrogen therapy is particularly good if you have a family history of osteoporosis or you yourself have osteoporosis currently. As was discussed in the chapter on osteoporosis, starting estrogen therapy as soon as you can after menopause will significantly help your bones and decrease your risk of fractures. If you have a strong family history of hip and spine fracture or many of your older relatives end up with a slouched spine in older age, you may consider estrogen therapy for prevention of these conditions.

STANDARD HORMONE FORMULATIONS

Estrogen only

Estradiol Tablets	Brand names: **Cenestin, Estrace, Femtrace, Menest, Ortho-Est,**	Good options for women without a uterus or with addition of progesterone for women who have a uterus
Estradiol Patches	Brand names: **Alora, Climara, Esclim, Menivelle, Vivelle-Dot**	Has the benefit of better absorption than oral options
Vaginal Estrogen	Brand names: **Estrace cream, Ogen cream, Vagifem tablets, Estring** vaginal ring	excellent for vaginal dryness and for bladder atrophy.
Synthetic Conjugated Estrogens	Brand names: **Cenestin, Enjuvia, Premarin, ESTRATEST** is the only precription estrogen with testosterone for women	Premarin Vaginal Cream is topical form

Estradiol Valerate and Estradiol Cypionate are the injectable forms done once a month

Estrogen and Progesterone Combinations

Estradiol and Progesterone Pills	Brand Names: **Activella, Angeliq, FemHrt, Prefes**t	excellent option, however, limited by number of dosing sizes
Estradiol and Progesterone Patches	Brand Names: **Combipatch, Climara Pro**	excellent options however, expensive and limited dosing amounts.
Conjugated Estrogen and Progesterone	**PremPro**	has more dosing sizes but is synthetic estrogen

Progesterone Only

Micronized Progesterone	Brand name **Prometrium**	My preferred progesterone but limited by only two dosing strengths. It is also used in compounded fromulations.
Medroxyprogesterone acetate	**Provera**	

COMPOUNDED HORMONE THERAPY

There are an infinite number of combinations since they are chosen for the patient. Here is an overview:

Estrogen alone	**Estradiol** (E2) alone or **estriol** (E3) alone	can be in oral, vaginal or topical forms
	Bi-estrogen usually in a ratio of 80 percent estriol with 20 percent estradiol; can also be made in a 50:50 ratio. **Tri-Estrogen** E3 80: E2 10 and Estrone 10 percent	oral, topical, vaginal or troche forms
Estrogen with progesterone	**Bi- and Tri-Estrogen with Prometrium**—See above with addition of 25-200 mg micronized progesterone	usually topical or pill form
Testosterone	**Testosterone** can be added to oral formulations but is not well absorbed. It is best as a topical gel in a dose of 2-12 mg.	Topicals can be dosed based on patient symptom relief
Progesterone	**Micronized progesterone** can be added to above treatments or made separately in a capsule or topical form. Used for perimenopause and estrogen excess syndromes	must be added to all estrogen therapy if a woman still has her uterus.

DHEA is a pre-hormone that may be added to boost one's natural production of hormones

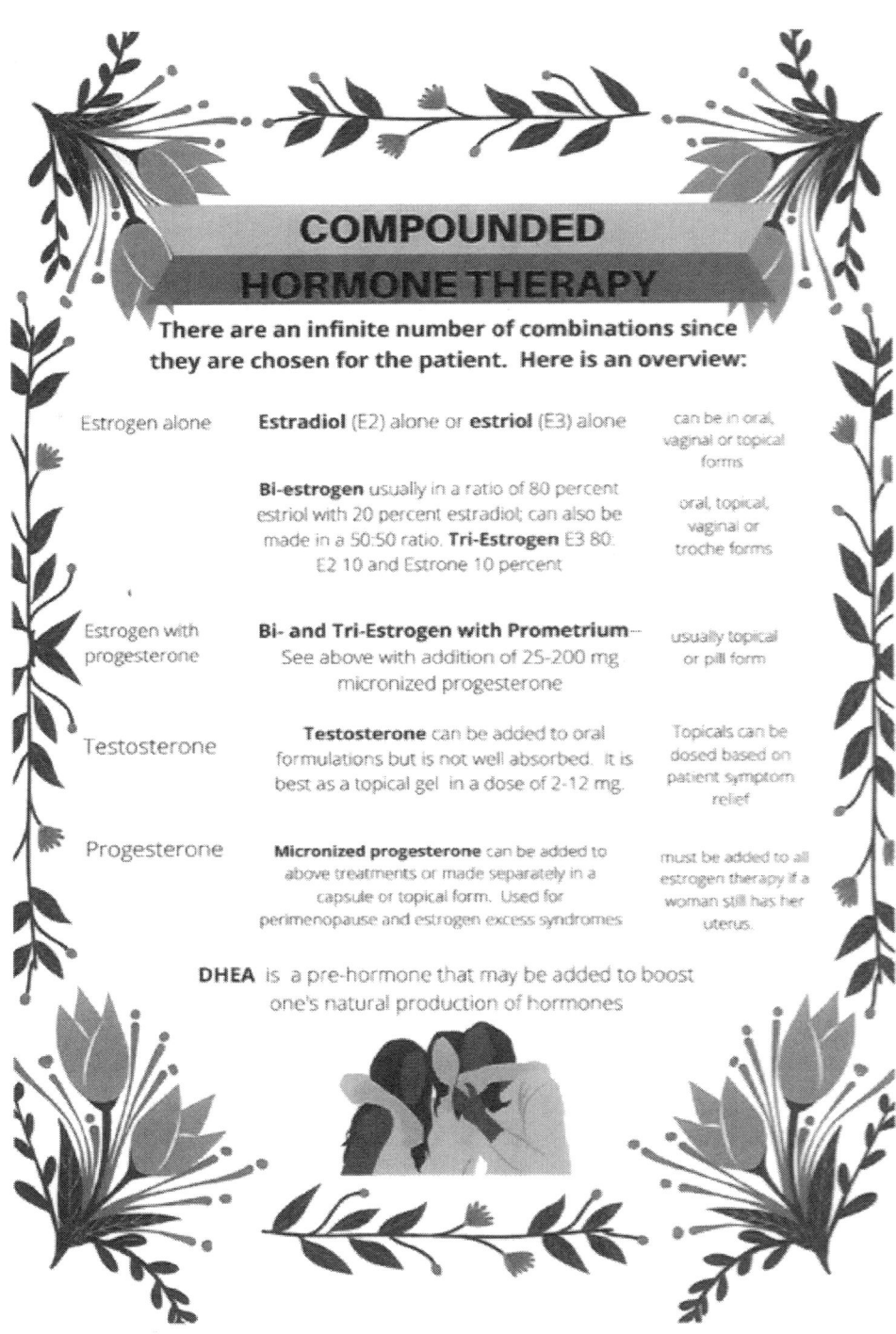

Chapter Ten: Non-Hormonal Treatment for Menopause

Some patients prefer to avoid hormones entirely for many reasons: they may have a history of breast cancer, be fearful of potential side effects of hormones or want to avoid prescriptions entirely. This chapter will introduce several options including non-hormonal prescriptions, herbals and other alternative treatments. Remember that if your symptoms are mild and not interfering with your day-to-day life, you may not have to take anything for menopause. Menopause is a natural life transition and many women stop having periods and have a few months of manageable symptoms that gradually go away as their bodies naturally withdraw from hormones and adjust to these changes. The options discussed in this chapter may be used short term to allow your body to make this transition with less symptoms resulting in better quality of life.

Standard Non-Hormonal Prescriptions

There are several non-hormonal prescriptions available used to control common symptoms of menopause. The most common medications prescribed by physicians are medications in the antidepressant class. This includes selective serotonin reuptake inhibitors (SSRI) like paroxetine (Paxil), fluoxetine (Prozac), sertraline (Zoloft), citalopram (Celexa) and selective serotonin and norepinephrine inhibitors (SSNRI) like venlafexine (Effexor). These are generally very effective for decreasing hot flashes and moodiness that accompany early menopause. Typically they are prescribed as a once-a-day dose and take effect in one to two weeks. They have the unfortunate side effects of weight gain (which has already been discussed as a common symptom of menopause) and decreased libido or sex drive. They can also interfere somewhat with falling asleep or staying asleep. Also, the first few days they are taken, people often have mild nausea, diarrhea, or constipation, which will gradually subside as the medication is continued. This symptom of nausea can be avoided by a gradual increase in the medication—taking half a pill a day for three days and then going back up to the full dose. Keep in mind that this class may trigger night sweats, another possible menopause symptom.

For women who mostly have difficulty falling asleep, using a tricyclic antidepressant like elavil or trazadone may be most effective. These medications also may help with hot flashes and moodiness, but primarily help a patient fall asleep and sleep through the night. For many women, proper sleep seems to improve the symptoms of irritability and mental fogginess, so emphasis on good sleep hygiene helps women suffering with menopausal symptoms. The above medications will be continued at least nine to 18 months until the brain and body have adjusted to a lower estrogen state, and then will be gradually tapered off to avoid the side effects of withdrawal such as dizziness.

Other medication options for hot flashes include several types of high blood pressure medications or anti-hypertensives. These include clonidine, verapamil and beta-blocker medications such as metoprolol or bisoprolol. Many of these can be taken once a day, and why they help hot flashes is unknown. If you are already on a blood pressure medication, you could choose to change to a type that may work better for hot flashes. Side effects of these medications are many and include decrease in blood pressure, fatigue, constipation and low heart rate. However, for many women these medications are very helpful at low doses for controlling hot flashes.

Less often prescribed options for hot flashes include pregabalin (Lyrica), and gabapentin (Neurontin). These are medications commonly used for pain, so if you suffer from arthritis in menopause these may have a combined effects of helping sleep, improving pain and decreasing hot flashes.

Herbal options

There is an amazing variety of herbal preparations that are very effective at helping women with many symptoms of menopause and perimenopause. Herbals preparation from plants produce chemicals that are very clean and specific to cellular receptors in our body. They do this by utilizing enzymatic reactions that make chemicals with a specific stereoisomer configuration versus multiple isomers as would occur in a chemical reaction in a pharmaceutical lab. These stereoisomers are chemicals that have identical composition but mirror each other in the arrangement of these molecules, much like our right and left hands, which are also "stereoisomers." Our bodies rely on chemicals that are a certain isomer, say only the "right-handed" configuration will work to unlock a cellular process. Potentially, herbals may be more potent with less side effects due to this characteristic. In addition, many of our prescription medications are actually made to replicate chemicals derived and isolated from plants.

Herbal options are also usually inexpensive and easy to obtain. Unfortunately, due to lack of funding for studies, many claims of symptom control or disease regulation often cannot be justified scientifically. Another concern with herbals is that we cannot be certain of potency or milligram amounts in each herbal brand or in each batch since they are not regulated quite as rigorously as prescriptions. However, there are European studies that substantiate claims of many herbal options. One reference that compiles this research is the The Complete German Commission E Monograph which is a compilation of European research done prior to the late 1970s on herbal preparations. A more recent publication is the PDR of Herbal Remedies, which includes references to the Commission E data.

Here a list of herbals that are commonly recognized as effective for some menopausal symptoms.

- **Black Cohosh** - This is a very effective herbal for hot flashes and is typically found in many combination herbal preparations such as Estroven, a brand of over-the-counter menopausal herbal. Effective doses vary according to potency of the herb. In general dosing ranges from 100-400 mg daily for help with hot flashes. Many women will use this for the first year or two after the start of menopause. It appears to also help with night sweats, brain fog, sleep and vaginal symptoms as well.

- **Evening Primrose Oil** - This oil is high in gamma-linoleic acid and has a mild progesterone-like effect. It can help with sleep, night sweats and hot flashes. The typical dose is 2-4 grams a day.

- **Natural progesterone cream** - These are usually made from wild yam into cream and also have a progesterone-like effect to help hot flashes. There are also some preparations that are made with USP progesterone such as that used in compounded formulations. It is important to check the expiration as creams have a shorter shelf life than other supplements. Typical doses are 40-200 mg daily.

- **Uva Ursi** - This herbal is used for help with the bladder, uterus and vaginal tissues and seems to promote vaginal lubrication and help with urinary symptoms such as increased urination or incontinence. Usual doses are 400-800 mg a day.

- **DHEA or dehydroepiandrosterone** - This is a precursor to our own natural sex hormones such as estrogen and testosterone. It is thought that adding it as a supplement may help your body make its own natural sex hormones. However, supplementing DHEA may suppress the adrenal glands, blunting natural production of DHEA. Also, if your ovaries are not longer functioning, then they will not convert the DHEA to estrogen and testosterone as they did premenopausal.

- **Dong Quai and Red Clover** - There is some antidotal evidence that these may be helpful for the transition to menopause. Often these preparations are not effective for hot flashes in patient.

- **Valarian Root** - A very helpful herbal for anxiousness, irritability and sleep.

- **St John's Wort** - Much like an antidepressant and has been studied in doses taken three times a day. It may help mental fogginess and hot flashes, irritability and sleep.

Alternative options for Treatment of Menopause

- **Acupuncture** - This option should be done with someone who is trained in traditional Chinese medicine, can be very effective for the transition through menopause. Acupuncture may work by providing feedback directly the thalamus and hypothalamus, which help the brain to coordinate pain pathways and hormonal integration as well as coordination of the parasympathetic and sympathetic systems. In other words, acupuncture may provide direct feedback and stimulation of centers in the brain. Regardless of its mechanism, acupuncture has been around for thousands of years and has been shown to be extremely effective for many conditions. With this modality, many patients get relief from hot flashes, mental fogginess, appetite changes and sleep disturbances. Usually it will take a series of sessions once a week or every other week for a four to six months to be effective. Since it is working on regulating your natural brain/body connection, there are few side effects.

- **Neurofeedback** - This is a procedure done by a trained counselor or therapist to help encourage certain brain wave patterns that are relaxing and improve focus. It can help with poor mood, memory and concentration as well as improve sleep and decrease anxiety. It generally takes 20 to 40 sessions to be affective. Neurofeedback also improves neuroplasticity or adaptation of the brain, which may be extremely helpful during menopause.

A word about sleep

Insomnia is a common complaint across all ages and sexes. It is particularly bad during menopause and contributes significantly to fatigue, concentration and mood during the day. Attention given to improving sleep will significantly improve quality of life. Good sleep hygiene involves creating a routine to suggest to your body that it is time to fall asleep at a certain time of day. This may involve a nice stretching routine while listening to relaxing music, a bath or reading a book. Meditation or breathing exercises even if for just a few minutes, help to tone the natural relaxation response prior to sleep. Herbals teas, crafts or watching the sunset may become part of your relaxation routine. Remember that this is a time to tune in to your body and your breath and to be accepting of your state at that moment, even if your brain is going a mile a minute. Become aware of the present, scan your body, and try to breath in relaxation and calmness. Alcohol may seem like it relaxes you at first, but is it very bad for sleep, often resulting in 2 am wakening and racing thoughts. Alcohol is a depressant and is extremely bad for those suffering from anxiety and depression. Keep in mind that a single cup of coffee may lessen duration of restorative sleep even 24-48 hours after a single cup. Also avoid any screens, like your cell phone and computer for 30 minutes prior to falling asleep. Menopause is a very important time to protect your sleep. It will help the rest of your body and mind during this transition.

We have introduced many options for management of menopause, hopefully it is not too overwhelming. Strategies can be tailored significantly to your particular situation. Don't be discouraged if one method does not work well for you. With a knowledgeable provider, you can discuss where one option has failed you and what symptoms are interfering most with your ability to work or fulfill your goals for a happy life. It may be a combination of strategies that will help you through. There is a light at the end of the tunnel when your body finally finds homeostasis with your hormonal level, whether it is with supplementation or letting your hormones remain at a naturally low level. In other words, your body will naturally become more predicable again within just a limited span of time—usually one to four years for most.

Chapter Eleven:
Putting It All Together,
An Intentional Living Plan

Nora Ephron
"Every so often I read a book about age, and whoever's writing it says it's great to be old. It's great to be wise and sage and mellow; it's great to be at the point where you understand just what matters in life. I can't stand people who say things like this." — *I Feel Bad About My Neck*, 2006

At 47 I had a wake up call forcing me to stop and examine my life: emergency surgery for appendicitis, which left me chronically fatigued with relentless migraine headaches for about six months. Believe me, there was no room in my life at that time for bed rest and naps. I had three kids—one in college, one a senior at high school and the other in middle school, each with their own very busy lives. I also ran a family practice office with my husband. I reluctantly gave myself a week to recover, still suffering daily from severe headaches, fatigue and fever. I had to go back to work; I already had a packed schedule of patients who had waited months for an appointment. The suffering continued for months, and I would wake up at night drenched in sweat, unable to go back to sleep. My hair was falling out and I felt anxious all the time. I sought the advice of many physicians who had different suggestions of what I could do to function better. I even started taking antidepressants without complete relief. Even as a doctor, I didn't know what was happening and who to turn to.

Finally I checked my blood work and on a whim decided to check for menopause with an FSH (follicle stimulating hormone) level— I was in menopause! I had stopped having periods many years prior due to a surgical procedure for heavy bleeding, so I hadn't realized that menopause was starting. I decided at that point to reexamine my life. Now was the time to slow down at work and take on less. I had always exercised regularly with running, but I incorporated yoga and strengthening for more relaxation and toning. I started hormones and drank less alcohol. I also turned to a counselor who helped me reevaluate my goals and dreams for the next phase of life. The fact that menopause had come at the busiest time of my life seemed overwhelming but it was also advantageous. It forced me to slow down and take a long survey of my health and life choices from an educated and wise perspective, freeing me to make new choices.

The advice in this book comes from my heart and from my experience as a doctor: ALL health and wellness fundamentally comes from a balanced diet and lifestyle. In this chapter, I would like to summarize a roadmap to longevity and quality of life as we age which includes changing habits and making healthy lifestyle modifications involving diet, exercise and meditation. To obtain a full and healthy life you will need to give daily attention to your diet, exercise, focused breathing exercises, establishing a support system of friends and family and continued attention on your long term goals and wishes. These are changes that you will strive to adhere to every day from now on, and not just a quick fix. Congratulations on making the first steps—this is a process and it will take some time to establish good habits as you age.

To help navigate this balance requires a relationship with a knowledgeable healthcare practitioner as your medical home coordinator. Enlisting the help of a nutritionist, personal trainer, naturopathic physician or mental health counselor can also be helpful. Get regular blood tests and exams with your primary provider rather than waiting until you have a long list of problems—your provider can then better focus on prevention and counseling rather than your immediate issues. If you are approaching menopause or already experiencing it, make sure you have on your team a practitioner knowledgeable about hormone management and female issues. You may find that due to health conditions, you will need to take medications. Be mindful of exactly what they are for, what the side effects may be and if there are interactions with other herbals or medications you may be taking.

Diet for Life

Your food makes up the building blocks of all of your body's cells; therefore, it is extremely important to have a good diet as you age. Overall it is best to consume a diet lower in carbohydrates, ideally around 125-150 grams of carbs a day. The addition of food high in omega-3 and 6 such as chia seeds, cold water fish and olive and flax oils is helpful for brain and heart health. Try to limit your sodium intake to less than 4000 mg a day for better blood pressure and decreased bloating and swelling. Avoid wheat, such as bread and pasta, as much as possible—it increases an inflammatory response and in the United States is highly processed with pesticides. Try to eat whole foods cooked at home so that you can control the amount of saturated fats and salt in your meal. Eat organic as much as you can, it is better for both your body and the planet. Add foods that are fermented and probiotic like kimchee, kombucha, yogurt, tempeh and miso for additional B12 benefits and to aid replenishing your intestinal micro-biome.

Should you take supplements? If you are mindful of a good diet, it may not be necessary. Supplements do provide extra insurance that you are getting optimal nutrition every day. Here is a list of commonly recommended supplements and benefits of each:

- **Probiotics** - This supplement is very beneficial to the immune system and gut health, especially for those who are recovering from leaky gut syndrome, who travel extensively, or who have taken antibiotics in the past. There is extensive research being done on specific strains for certain conditions but the science is still in the early stages. It is best to take a broad spectrum probiotic that contains acidophilus, bifidbactum and lactobacillus, at least 10 million CFUs. Also, feed your good microbiome with high fiber foods, such as vegetables and whole grains.

- **Vitamin B complex** - These are easily cooked out of foods but are essential for cellular metabolism. B12 in particular has complicated absorption made worse with aging, resulting in the need for vitamin B12 shots for some people. Recommend amount is 1000 mcg of B-12 a day.

- **Omega 3,6 supplements** - These fatty acids are not made in our bodies and must be obtained from our diet. Recommended amount is 1-2 grams a day.

- **Vitamin D3** - This drop or capsule is important for bone health and calcium absorption and may be protective to our neurological system. Recommended amount is 2000-4000 IU daily.

- **Magnesium** - This is a fantastic mineral found in green leafy vegetables and is in the very center of the chlorophyll molecule in plants involved in photosynthesis. We are probably meant to get a larger quantity of green leafy vegetables than we do in a modern diet, so supplementation is necessary. It has many benefits including help with sleep, muscle relaxation, increased bowel movements. It helps prevent migraines and cramping with periods. It is used in the hospital intravenously for treatment of pre-eclampsia in pregnancy which involves high blood pressure, seizures and leg swelling, so it may have a benefit to lowering blood pressure as well in a non-pregnancy state. The usual dose is 200-600 mg a day.

Exercise

If only we continued to play as much as we did as kids, getting plenty of exercise outside with friends. Instead many of us find ourselves sitting for very long hours each day at a computer or in the car as we get older. Because of this tendency towards a sedentary lifestyle, we need to incorporate exercise to keep our muscles, heart and lungs strong. This may be less structured, such as getting 5000-10,000 steps a day on a step counter or organized classes. You get to decide, so pick something that gives you pleasure that you can stick with—it doesn't need to be running your first marathon! Best practice is to exercise 30-60 minutes a day, five days a week and spend at least 30 minutes three days a week doing weight bearing exercise. Exercise helps keep your bones from being prone to breaking, decreases risk of falling, and increases your metabolism. It also makes you less prone to falling as you age. Here are some suggestions:

Outdoor activities
walking, running, hiking
climbing
biking/mountain biking
gardening/yard work

Winter sports
nordic ski
cross country ski

Team Sports
tennis
golfing
pickle ball
soccer
baseball/softball

Water sports
kayaking
swimming
surfing
snorkeling/scuba diving
rowing/canoeing/paddle

Gym activities
weight lifting spin class
hula hoop
yoga
pilates
cross-fit
gymnastics

Dance Class
line dancing
zumba
ballet
African dance

Martial Arts
judo
aikido
karate

The list goes on and on. Just think of whether you may like an organized activity or team sport for the social aspect, or would rather have something you do at your own pace. Remember that there are many classes available online as well, easily accessed on YouTube, or an application of something you may be interested in such as yoga or dance.

Exercise done outside has the additional benefit of making you focus on the present moment and gives you the opportunity to notice the beauty in which we live. This is remarkably good for mood and for relaxation. In Japan, it is called "forest bathing" and in 1982 was recommended nationally to help decrease stress levels of people living in more urban settings. If you are enjoying traveling more as you age, take the opportunity to seek out local trails and forests in the countries you are exploring for a whole new dimension in local lifestyle. Or better yet, explore our many national parks with thousands of acres of protected lands, trails, rivers and lakes.

Focused Breathing or Meditation

Our nervous system has two automatic systems called the parasympathetic and sympathetic systems. They work together always like a yin/yang with one system having a higher "tone" or being more active in a given situation. The parasympathetic system is important during times of rest and rejuvenation, promoting good digestion, sleep and repair of damage that may have occurred during a normal day. The sympathetic system is important for "fight or flight," being active when it is time to act, raising our heart rate and focus so that we can avoid danger.

In our society, we are rewarded with increased income for working hard, with sometimes long, stressful hours. We promote this in our children, organizing days that are completely filled with activities, school and chores. This habit at an early age encourages chronic stimulation of the the sympathetic (fight or flight) system in an effort to get ahead. Social media and hand-held computers may make this worse, encouraging us to be constantly engaged in current events and what our friends are doing, promoting a feeling of anxiety. It is well known, even in medical literature, that chronic stress directly relates to increased disease.

It is nearly impossible to talk ourselves out of being less stressed. Luckily, there is much research that suggests that focused breathing, even for two to ten minutes a day, can be very helpful to increasing parasympathetic tone (the relaxation system), thereby increasing your natural relaxation response. You can do this simply by breathing slowly for two minutes with your eyes closed. In addition there are many meditation techniques that have been around for hundreds of years, such those found in buddhism or yogic traditions. In the past few years, many computer or phone apps such as Headspace or Calm have been developed that help the user stimulate the relaxation response through breathing. Finding one that works for you that you can do daily, is the key. Meditation or mindfulness breathing also has the benefit of helping you separate from your thought and grounding you in the present moment, which is truly where life is happening. In the words of John Lennon, "Life is what happens to you while you are busy making other plans." Whether life is slowing down or staying just as busy as always for you, find a way to incorporate this important tool.

Here is a Simple Meditation Technique:

- Sit comfortably in a chair or cross legged on the floor.

- Start by taking a few deep breaths.

- Focus your attention to the top of your head; try to keep your attention there as much as possible.

- Use a mantra that you will repeat in the same pattern as your breathing. For example you can repeat to yourself "I am the light" or "I am peace." When you inhale think "I am" and when you breath out think "the light."

- Continue this way for 10-15 minutes. You may get off track by thinking of other things, but this is normal. Just go back to focusing on the top of your head and your mantra each time.

The change will be gradual and subtle for most. Eventually you will notice there are times when you are sitting without having the constant chatter of thoughts. You may notice more times of day that you are relaxed as you are in mindful breathing. This is the goal. Try not to get too frustrated when you have thoughts, you want to get in touch with the relaxed part of you that is observing your thoughts. It takes practice.

Try to do this every day if possible.

Find Your Tribe

Many of us have heard about research and publications commending the lifestyles of those living in the Mediterranean due to the longevity that is found on many island countries in that region. Much attention has been given to the diet of those people suggesting that we should all consume more fish, olive oil, wine and vegetables to live longer. However, more recent studies done on increasing intake of olive oil and wine since this theory has come out have not completely supported that longevity for Mediterraneans is just from diet. There have been some suggestions that perhaps it is their lifestyle beyond eating that actually promotes longevity for the Mediterranean people. It has been suggested, for example, those living on the island of Crete usually live in smaller communities where there is much social interaction, including morning breaks to talk, and long afternoon lunches. They take time to savor their food and will be mindful while they are eating. If there is something on your land that needs upkeep, neighbors will pitch in and help. In conclusion, it appears that this attention to supporting each other may actually be the most important variable to promoting longevity.

Another example of this is seen in cancer patients. It has been scientifically proven that people with cancer live longer on average when they take the time to attend support groups for their illness. There is something emotionally supportive about connecting with others, either lending an ear and offering support or having the extra security that someone has your back that makes us actually live longer. No one is certain the biological basis for this, but it appears to be very powerful.

As we age we are faced with the loss of family members and friends and we experience changes in our careers and places where we live. Finding people in the area that you live to help lend a hand when you are in need is important. This may be in your neighborhood, in your church or religious group, a volunteer organization, organized sports, art or singing groups or staying connected with family. Find a way to connect with those around you. You are worth it and have a great deal to contribute in wisdom and insight to the planet. Find your tribe of people who foster this in you so you can make the most of the next 50 years.

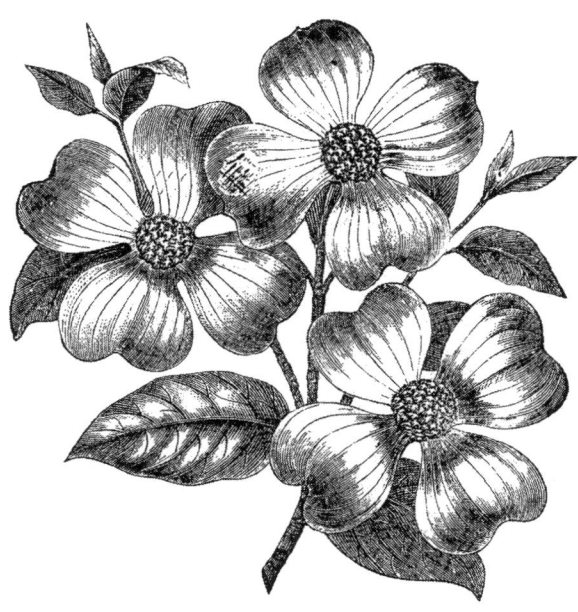

Works Cited and Additional Reading

Blumenthal, Mark. Herbal Medicine: Expanded Commision E Monographs. Integrative Medicine Communications, 2000.

Carroll, Judith E., et al. "Epigenetic Aging and Immune Senescence in Women With Insomnia Symptoms: Findings from the Women's Health Initiative Study." Biological Psychiatry, vol. 81, no. 2, 2017, pp. 136–144., doi:10.1016/j.biopsych.2016.07.008.

Christensen, Margaret. "Reducing Chronic Disease Risk at Menopause Using Nutrition." The Institute for Functional Medicine, 17 Dec. 2019, www.ifm.org/functional-medicine/.

Crandall, Carolyn J., et al. "Safety of Vaginal Estrogens." Menopause, vol. 27, no. 3, 2020, pp. 339–360., doi:10.1097/gme.0000000000001468.

Desai, Maunil K., and Roberta Diaz Brinton. "Autoimmune Disease in Women: Endocrine Transition and Risk Across the Lifespan." Frontiers in Endocrinology, vol. 10, 2019, doi:10.3389/fendo.2019.00265.

Geller, Stacie E., and Laura Studee. "Contemporary Alternatives to Plant Estrogens for Menopause." Maturitas, vol. 55, 2006, doi:10.1016/j.maturitas.2006.06.012.

Heo, Young-A. "Prasterone: A Review in Vulvovaginal Atrophy." Drugs & Aging, vol. 36, no. 8, 2019, pp. 781–788., doi:10.1007/s40266-019-00693-6.

Kanherkar, Riya R., et al. "Epigenetics across the Human Lifespan." Frontiers in Cell and Developmental Biology, vol. 2, 2014, doi:10.3389/fcell.2014.00049.

Kapoor, Ekta, et al. "Weight Gain in Women at Midlife: A Concise Review of the Pathophysiology and Strategies for Management." Mayo Clinic Proceedings, vol. 92, no. 10, 2017, pp. 1552–1558., doi:10.1016/j.mayocp.2017.08.004.

Kozakowski, Jarosław, et al. "Obesity in Menopause – Our Negligence or an Unfortunate Inevitability?" Menopausal Review, vol. 2, 2017, pp. 61–65., doi:10.5114/pm.2017.68594.

Krysiak, Robert, et al. "The Effect of Gluten-Free Diet on Thyroid Autoimmunity in Drug-Naïve Women with Hashimoto's Thyroiditis: A Pilot Study." Experimental and Clinical Endocrinology & Diabetes, vol. 127, no. 07, 2018, pp. 417–422., doi:10.1055/a-0653-7108.

Pharmacists, staff. "Female Hormone Therapy Options." Women's International Pharmacy, 26 Aug. 2020, www.womensinternational.com/.

Talsania, Mitali, and Robert Hal Scofield. "Menopause and Rheumatic Disease." Rheumatic Disease Clinics of North America, vol. 43, no. 2, 2017, pp. 287–302., doi:10.1016/j.rdc.2016.12.011.

Traish, Abdulmaged M., et al. "Role of Androgens in Female Genitourinary Tissue Structure and Function: Implications in the Genitourinary Syndrome of Menopause." Sexual Medicine Reviews, vol. 6, no. 4, 2018, pp. 558–571., doi:10.1016/j.sxmr.2018.03.005.

Wang, Yiwei, et al. "(PDF) Transitions in Metabolic and Immune Systems from Pre ..." Transitions in Metabolic and Immune Systems from Pre-Menopause to Post-Menopause: Implications for Age-Associated Neurodegenerative Disease, 2020.

Wickman, Julie m. "Androgen Therapy in Women." U.S. Pharmacist, 20 Aug. 2014.

Writing Group for The Women's Health Initiative Investigators, . "Risks and Benefits of Estrogen Plus Progestin in Healthy Postmenopausal Women: Principal Results From the Women's Health Initiative Randomized Controlled Trial." JAMA: The Journal of the American Medical Association, vol. 288, no. 3, 2002, pp. 321-333., doi:10.1001/jama.288.3.321.

Glossary

Bioidentical hormones - This is a prescription that may be in cream, pellet, capsule or sublingual form, also known as "natural hormones" or "compounded hormones". It is typically made in a specialized pharmacy in which pharmacists are trained to synthesize prescriptions.

Corpus luteum - The shell of an egg that is produced in the ovary and will secrete the hormone progesterone.

DNA (genes) - This chemical structure is found in the in nearly every cell and contained the inherited code or blueprint for the entire body. It may contain certain mutations or changes can result in cancer. Currently, there is available testing for determining a persons entire genetic code or sequence.

Epigenetics - The study of changes in the body due to the how genes are expressed or turned on. This may be due to numerous factors including, but not limited to, environment, aging, diseases or stress.

Estrogen - A hormone typically produced in women in the ovaries and causes female development and menstruation

Follicular phase - This typically the first 14 days of a menstrual cycle when the egg is developing in the ovary and secreting estrogen. It terminates when the egg follicle breaks open and releases the egg into the fallopian tube.

Formulary - This is a catalogue of medications, and commonly refers to those prescriptions covered by an insurance company and the tiers of cost to the insured patient. Compounded hormones are usually not included in most formularies.

FSH/LH - Hormones that are produced the pituitary gland located in the brain to stimulate the ovaries to ovulate. They are highest during ovulation and during menopause. This value can be checked to confirm menopause.

Insulin - A hormones that is made in the pancreas located in the stomach are that will control blood sugar. In type one diabetes it is not produced and in type two diabetes it is too high. It may stimulate the ovary to produced cyst in PCOS (polycystic ovarian syndrome).

Luteal phase: - The last 14 days of a menstrual cycle in which the corpus luteum is making large amounts of progesterone, resulting in stimulation of the uterine lining. At the end of the phase is a menstrual period.

Menopause - This is when the ovaries stop making eggs and hormones. It can also occur surgically when the ovaries are removed during a hysterectomy. Typically we consider a woman to be post-menopausal when they have gone an entire year without a period.

Menstrual cycle - The monthly cycle of hormonal changes that cause a period in a female, usually lasting 25-28 days.

Ovary - There are usually two of these glands located on either side of the uterus and are responsible for making an egg. A fertilized egg will then develop into an embryo.

Perimenopause - The time prior to complete cessation of periods which does not have a particular timespan and typically starts in one's forties. There can be large fluctuations of hormones during this time and irregular periods.

Progesterone - A hormone made in the luteal phase responsible for stimulating the uterine lining.

Pituitary gland - A polyp like brain structure that secretes multiple hormones to stimulate various glands in the body. This includes the ovaries, breasts, adrenal glands and thyroid. It is also called the "master gland".

Standard pharmacy - This may be a local pharmacy or mail in pharmacy that will fill prescriptions that are made by large pharmaceutical companies.

Uterus - A female organ located in the pelvis that will hold a pregnancy. It contains fallopian tubes that connect to the ovaries and a cervix that is the opening to the vagina.

Made in the USA
Coppell, TX
10 April 2024

31122663R00055